Swollen, Bloated and Puffy

A MANUAL LYMPHATIC DRAINAGE THERAPIST'S GUIDE TO REDUCING SWELLING IN THE FACE AND BODY

KATHLEEN LISSON CMT, CLT

All Rights Reserved © copyright:2017 Kathleen Lisson. First Printing: 2017. No portion of this book may be copied, retransmitted, reposted, duplicated, or otherwise used without the express written approval of the author, except by reviewers who may quote brief excerpts in connection with a review.

United States laws and regulations are public domain and not subject to copyright. Any unauthorized copying, reproduction, translation, or distribution of any part of this material without permission by the author is prohibited and against the law.

Disclaimer and Terms of Use

No information contained in this book should be considered as medical advice. Your reliance upon information and content obtained by you at or through this publication is solely at your own risk. Solace Massage and Mindfulness or the author assumes no liability or responsibility for damage or injury to you, other persons, or property arising from any use of any product, information, idea, or instruction contained in the content or services provided to you through this book. Reliance upon information contained in this material is solely at the reader's own risk. The author has no financial interest in and receive no compensation from manufacturers of products or websites mentioned in this book.

ISBN-13: 978-1548415433

ISBN-10: 154841543X

TABLE OF CONTENTS

Introduction .... *v*

PART 1 – WHAT IS LYMPHATIC MASSAGE?
Chapter 1: How to Have a Happy Lymphatic System 3

PART 2 – HOW TO REDUCE SWELLING
Chapter 2: What to Put On and In Your Face and
Body to Reduce Swelling 13

Chapter 3: What to Wear to Reduce Swelling 33

Chapter 4: Let's Use Gravity and our Muscles to Reduce Swelling 39

Chapter 5: How to Use Breathing to Boost your Lymphatic System 47

PART 3 – LET'S HAVE A WOMAN TO WOMAN TALK ABOUT CONSTIPATION AND INCONTINENCE
Chapter 6: Bonus Chapter for Mothers and all Ladies over 40 55

Another BONUS: Have you Heard of This? &
Why am I Swollen There? 67

PART 4 – YOUR IMMUNE SYSTEM
Chapter 7: Worried Sick – How to Improve your Immune System 73

Chapter 8: Seven Tips for Boosting Your Mood and Reducing Stress 109

Chapter 9: If You are Nervous Before Surgery 113

Conclusion *119*

Bibliography *125*

About the Author *135*

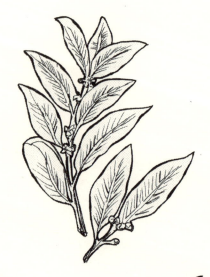

Bay Laurel

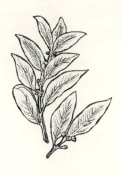

INTRODUCTION

Hello, my name is Kathleen Lisson. I live in San Diego, but my first adult experience with swelling happened on the side of a ski slope in Western Massachusetts. I was in my late thirties and had gone skiing to get out of the house after a particularly insane breakup with a boyfriend. I was on a 'green' hill, taking my time, and skied over to the side to let the lady behind me pass me by. I saw her coming, coming, coming and SMASH. She hit me on my right side and I crumpled to the ground. Managing to get back up and reluctant to make her feel even worse after her repeated apologies, I told her I was OK and to keep on skiing. I got up and tried to make it down the hill, but within a minute my right eye swelled shut. Long story short, I was rescued by the ski patrol, strapped onto a toboggan, hauled down the mountain, and driven by a friend to the local ER in my town later that day. The verdict: my right cheekbone was shattered and I needed reconstructive surgery.

Thanks to Dr. Stephane Braun, my surgery was successful, but when it rains, it pours – in the next decade I sprained my right ankle and had Mohs surgery on my face to remove skin cancer. The one thing all these incidents had in common? Swelling. Unsightly facial swelling that affected my ability to return to my career in the public eye as a PR rep, ankle and foot swelling that affected my ability to pursue my passion of long distance running, and swelling under my eye after cancer surgery that affected my enjoyment of reading. In every instance I was told the swelling was normal and that the best thing to do was to wait patiently for my body to heal itself.

What did you just say? You've heard that from your doctor, too? We're not alone. Doc is right, swelling is a normal part of recovery from trauma as well as plastic, reconstructive and orthopedic surgery, but there ARE ways to reduce swelling and heal faster.

Why did I write this book?

We connected with one another because you have swelling, too. Board Certified Plastic Surgeons and Naturopaths refer their clients to me to reduce the heavy, tight feeling that swelling can bring. Many of my clients fall asleep during their treatments and I take this as a compliment! It means they feels safe and have given me their trust.

When I provide manual lymphatic drainage massage I get to hear my client's stories and talk with them about their concerns. Some want to 'detox' to banish puffiness and stop bloating and abdominal distention. Others have recently had surgery or an injury and want to reduce swelling, or have had lymphedema or lipedema for years and are looking for some new tips on reducing edema. The one comment I hear more than anything else when I talk to people about my profession is — "I wish I knew this existed," whether it was when they were facing surgery, when their mother or other loved one had cancer (I also have training in oncology and scar massage) or when they were struggling with swelling in the weeks and months after trauma or an operation.

In this booklet I will share with you my top tips picked up from my training as a Certified Lymphedema Therapist, conversations with Surgeons and Physical Therapists, presentations at lymphedema conferences and tips shared by ladies with lymphedema and lipedema sharing what has worked best for them. Many of the tips are backed by research. I will even share a few more 'interesting' ways to reduce swelling and boost your immune system!

First, let's learn a little bit about our body's lymphatic system and what to expect after your manual lymphatic drainage session. If you have had a massage session with me, you know how excited I get about our lymphatic system. I find it fascinating and hope you will, too.

Important Note: the tips discussed in this book were compiled through reviewing research studies and published literature on lymphedema and lipedema, interviewing experts on swelling reduction and stress-busting techniques, and listening to clients suffering

Swollen, Bloated and Puffy

with swelling first-hand. Experts may disagree and scientific advances may render some of this information outdated. The author assumes no responsibility for any outcome of applying the information in this book for self-care. If you have any safety-related questions about the application of techniques discussed in this booklet, please consult your physician or plastic surgeon.

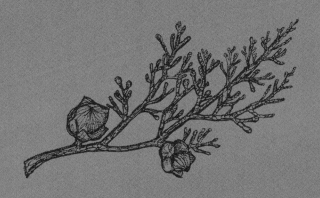

PART 1

WHAT IS LYMPHATIC MASSAGE?

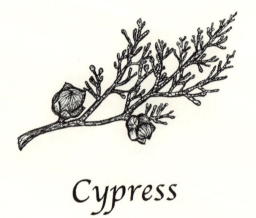

Cypress

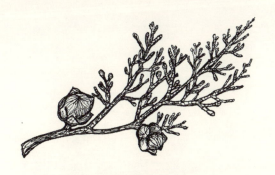

CHAPTER 1

HOW TO HAVE A HAPPY LYMPHATIC SYSTEM

The lymphatic system works with our body's circulatory system and is a part of our body's immune system. Let's begin by reviewing what we know about the circulatory system. The blood carries the nourishment that our cells need to thrive – blood leaves the heart and travels first in our arteries, then to the capillaries and finally through the capillary wall to each and every cell. Capillaries are permeable, so the nutrients the cells need are pushed from the blood in the capillary to the area around the cells. The fluids bathing the cells are called interstitial fluids, because they are 'inter' or between the cells. The cells take what they need and also dispose of all their waste products into this fluid. The blood in our venules recollects the majority of the waste products from the interstitial fluid and brings them back via the veins to the heart, then the lungs, liver and kidneys for processing and disposal.

Here's something I never learned in high school biology — about 2 liters of the fluids our cells no longer need each day do not go directly back into the veins. This fluid, which includes protein and fat molecules, waste products and water, is instead carried back to the heart through the lymphatic system. The lymphatic system is a network of tiny tubes that filters this fluid with the help of lymph nodes before returning it to rejoin the bloodstream at a point just above the heart.

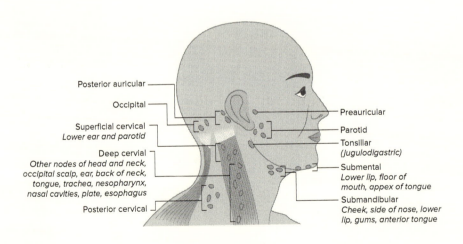

Swollen, Bloated and Puffy

Chapter 1: How to Have a Happy Lymphatic System

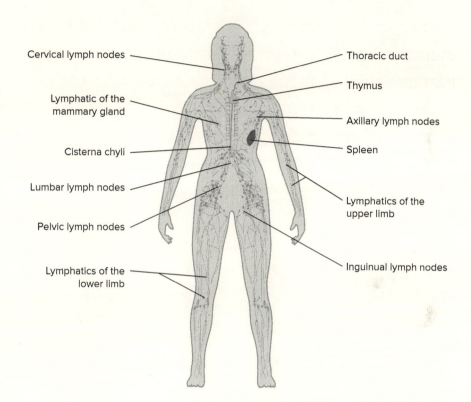

You may have heard of lymph nodes – they are an important part of our immune system. I can feel the lymph nodes in my neck get larger when I am feeling under the weather. If you have a bout of diarrhea a half hour after every time you eat high fat foods like cream or a hamburger, it's a warning sign that the abdominal lymphatics are not functioning effectively. Our lymphocytes, or white blood cells, are present in

Swollen, Bloated and Puffy

our lymph nodes and identify and respond to microbes and cancer cells when they 'find' them in the lymphatic fluid. I explain why every session starts with neck and abdomen work to all my new clients – it's because many of our body's 600 – 700 lymph nodes are found in our intestines, head and neck. This makes sense because the body needs to filter and respond to potential pathogens from the food we eat and potential threats sneaking in at the other entrances of the body – our eyes, ears, nose and mouth.

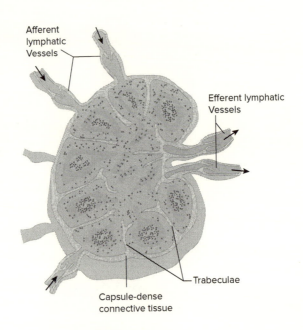

How can we help our lymph system function? Most healthy people don't need to worry too much about their lymphatic system. We may get a little puffy when eating the wrong foods, drinking alcohol or exercising in hot weather, but the swelling goes down on its own. When the body is compromised, our lymphatic system may need a boost. Orthopedic, plastic and reconstructive surgery – and even a C-section – can result in persistent swelling around the incision area. A condition called secondary lymphedema can occur if lymph nodes are removed or harmed during cancer treatment that results in swelling of an arm, leg, face or neck. Many cases of primary lymphedema are present at birth or become visible while the patient is young, and occur as a result of genes or other causes. I have training and expertise to use manual lymphatic drainage to help reduce swelling in each of these cases.

There are several ways to help the lymphatic system, including:

- Diaphragmatic (belly) breathing
- Exercising and muscle movement – especially the calves

- External pressure (immersion in water or wearing bandaging and compression garments) and
- Utilization of an external compression technique like Manual Lymphatic Drainage

Manual lymphatic drainage is a light pressure massage technique that stimulates the lymphatic system to carry extra fluid and filter that fluid through our lymph nodes before returning it to the heart. Manual lymphatic drainage reduces the 'tight or heavy' feeling that swelling brings after surgery and is also used to treat lymphedema that results from many types of cancer treatment, including treatment for head & neck as well as breast and gynecological cancer.

What to Expect After Your Manual Lymphatic Drainage Massage

These tips are what every one of my clients hears after their massage.

I worked first on your abdomen and neck to encourage your lymphatic system to start working at an increased rate. Then I massaged the lymph nodes in the armpits or the hips, whichever was closer to your area of swelling. Then, using soft, skin stretching strokes, I encouraged the flow of lymph away from the swollen area and into the lymphatic system so it could return to the heart. If you had surgery, I used 'anastamoses,' or cross-connections, to reroute lymph fluid away from the incision site to adjacent parts of your lymphatic system. The lymphatic system will keep on working hard to remove swelling as best it can for a period of time after the massage. For best results, use bandages or compression garments if you have them and put them on as soon as possible after the MLD treatment. Relaxation and elevation of the swollen area can also help boost lymphatic flow.

Please drink plenty of water! Water is essential for your body. Reducing water intake will NOT reduce swelling.

You may urinate more as you body reduces the swelling in the affected area and you may become less constipated as a result of the deep abdominal work that was part of your treatment. Later in this booklet I will share other techniques that may make you more 'regular.'

Swollen, Bloated and Puffy

Just like the hints and tips I share later in the book, manual lymphatic drainage massage is not a silver bullet or a quick fix. Your swelling will not be completely resolved in only one session. Many detox programs sell themselves as a miracle cure for all types of illness. Manual lymphatic drainage works with your body to improve the flow of lymph, no more and no less.

So, now we know what the lymphatic system is and what it does. How can we help a healthy lymphatic system? Read on to find out.

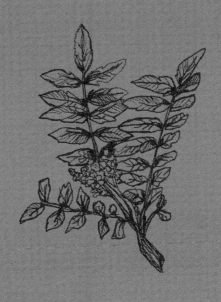

PART 2
HOW TO REDUCE SWELLING

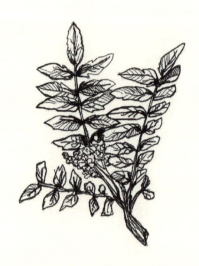

Frankincense

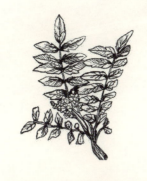

CHAPTER 2

WHAT TO PUT ON AND IN YOUR FACE AND BODY TO REDUCE SWELLING

Our skin is our body's biggest organ and our protection and defense system. Our skin can also offer us information about what is happening inside our body. How? Just look in the mirror and see what your skin is telling you. Do you have a healthy glow or a dull, swollen face and body? Because our skin is giving us clues as to the health of our body, the best long-term cure is to improve our overall health, not just seek a quick fix or cover it with makeup to hide our imperfections. Having skin cancer has inspired me to take better care of my skin and use my skin to gauge how healthy I am. My top three recommendations for clients who have recently undergone surgery:

- If you are curious whether a product will work for you, test it on a small patch of skin. Don't use a popular skin product if your skin doesn't like it. Let your skin be the judge, not the beauty blogger on YouTube or Instagram
- If you have recently had facial surgery, only use products you have used before and do not use wipes to clean your face as they can pull on the skin
- If you have an open wound or incision from a recent surgery, get your doctor's OK before you try the following tips near your surgery site

If your skin is not sensitive to any of the ingredients in the following treatments, try them out and see if they help reduce your swelling.

Essential Oils for Balancing the Body's Lymphatic System

First, a word (or about 500) about essential oil safety. As a Certified Aromatherapist, I get asked all the time what brand of essential oils I use. I agree that it is hard to separate fact from hype because many of the voices on the internet giving advice on essential oils are salespeople. I am not affiliated with any company and I do not make any profit off of recommending or selling essential oils.

Essential oils and aromatic botanicals have been around for thousands of years, but the past decade has seen increased interest and availability of these strongly scented oils in tiny little colored bottles. When in the space of a few months last year I saw that:

- A tummy tuck client was using lavender essential oil to control her pain after her plastic surgery
- A lymphedema client was using geranium to boost her lymphatic system and
- My brother's wife was diffusing oils to calm my family while on vacation

I knew that I had to seek out college-level training on the effects of Aromatherapy in order to get the facts about essential oils and better serve you and my other clients.

Essential oils can be used with water in a diffuser and inhaled, with paraben-free lotion or oil and massaged on the skin and with water in a spray bottle as a mist for linens and on the body. What do all of these have in common? In each instance, if the oil is going to be in contact with the body, the essential oil is NOT used without first diluting it. I was shocked when I heard a woman selling essential oils recommend that people in her workshop apply them directly to the skin. I was even more dismayed when she claimed that the burning feeling that some felt was an indication that it was 'working.' If anything you put on your skin results in a burning sensation, it is your body telling you it is being injured, not healed. I only use essential oils straight from the bottle if I am placing a few drops in an essential oil necklace or on a handkerchief and smelling the aroma a few inches away from my body.

So, now that I've said my piece on how to use them safely, how can we use essential oils? In the wonderful book *Eat Drink Heal*, Plastic Surgeon Gregory A. Buford recommends a combination of vitamins, minerals, supplements, foods and stress reduction techniques, including aromatherapy, to prepare the body for

Swollen, Bloated and Puffy

surgery. The text emphasizes that each of the following essential oils should NOT be used straight, but added to a base of grape seed, almond or apricot seed oil. Dr. Buford shares that his colleague, board-certified anesthesiologist Dr. Nancy Thurman's recommended essential oils for calming the body and mind before surgery include lavender, rose and geranium. Dr. Thurman also recommends using citrus aromas after surgery and peppermint (Mentha piperita), spearmint (Mentha spicata) and ginger (Zingiber officinale) to control nausea in the recovery room (Buford 2016).

Aromatherapist Salvatore Battaglia is the author of *The Complete Guide to Aromatherapy*. His recommended essential oils for improved lymphatic function include citrus oils, peppermint (Mentha piperita), rosemary (Rosemarinus officinalis) and geranium (Pelargonium graveolens) essential oils. A few drops can be added to a palmful of paraben free body lotion and applied to the skin. Take care to protect skin from sun exposure, as citrus oils can increase the chances of sun damage (Battaglia 2003).

Linda-Anne Kahn is a Clinical Aromatherapist, Certified Lymphedema Therapist, co-author of the book *Lymphedema and Lipedema Nutrition Guide* and owner of the Beauty Kliniek spa in San Diego. She specializes in the treatment of Lymphedema, Lipedema and Dercum's disease. Linda-Anne shares information about several essential oils that balance and harmonize the lymphatic system on her spa's blog. Her recommended essential oils include angelica root (Angelica archangelica) bay laurel (Laurus nobilis), bergamot (Citrus bergamia), cedar (Cedrus atlantica), cypress (Cupressus sempervirens) grapefruit (Citrus paradisi), juniper berry (Juniperus communis), lemon (Citrus limon) and sweet orange (Citrus Sinensis). Linda-Anne sells a lymphatic blend from her spa's aromatherapy line Varenya Essentials called 'Flow' which contains grapefruit, cypress, lemon and rosemary essential oils (Kahn, n.d.).

Integrative Cardiologist Mimi Guarneri shares her essential oil picks for making one's home into "a sanctuary for your soul" in her book *108 Pearls to Awaken Your Healing Potential*. Dr. Guarneri suggests trying lavender, jasmine and geranium and calls lavender "one of nature's most relaxing scents." She also suggests placing fresh lavender in the bedroom or growing night blooming jasmine or gardenias by the bedroom window (Guarneri, 2017).

The 2014 *Evidence-Based Complementary and Alternative Medicine* journal article 'Essential Oils for Complementary Treatment of Surgical Patients: State of the Art' by Susanna Stea provides an overview of research on the effect of lavender (Lavandula angustifolia, Lavandula stoechas, Lavandula latifolia, Lavandula intermedia), orange (Citrus sinensis) and peppermint (Mentha piperita) essential oils to reduce anxiety and pain and offers mixed evidence (Stea, 2014). You'll find references at the end of this booklet to this research as well as the other articles and books I mention in this text.

Keep in mind that the FDA does not regulate essential oils as a medicine and I am not a doctor so I cannot diagnose or treat any disease. Experimentation is the best way to determine which essential oil your body likes the most, and spending a few hours smelling different essential oils can be a fun and relaxing experience!

Add a list of your favorite Essential Oils here:

_____

_____

_____

What Else Can I Use, Kathleen?

My vision for this section of the booklet is to provide a list of swelling-reduction tips you can use over and over again and share with family and friends. Let's take a playful look at the advice I've collected from experts, clients and other ladies dealing with swelling! I encourage you (with your doctor's permission) to experiment and see which tips work best for you. Before you try anything special, make sure you've mastered the basics to helping your body heal – following your physician or plastic surgeon's orders, eating healthy and not smoking.

The following techniques work by reducing the amount of blood our body pumps to the treated area.

Swollen, Bloated and Puffy

Reducing blood flow will reduce the amount of fluid the lymphatic system has to move back to the heart. This is similar to the traditional advice to apply ice to an injury to reduce swelling.

Gel Masks or Face Masks

Aah, there is nothing better for my sinus headaches or after a night of drinking or too little sleep than to stumble to the fridge and slip a cool face mask over my puffy eyes and face! I like the Ikisdo Care face mask from Amazon. My husband is used to seeing me cooking eggs in a face mask at seven in the morning after a late night.

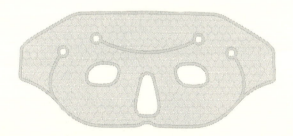

Face Rollers

Remember 2015, when all the beauty magazines and bloggers discovered face rollers? They are still around, a little cheaper now, and still work to reduce puffiness in the face. I store my face rollers in the freezer, right next to those Cornish Hens my husband wanted me to order from Amazon Fresh a few months ago.

My main everyday facial swelling problem is puffy eyelids. The first roller I use is about as wide as my hand and works well for waking me up if I didn't get enough sleep the night before. It's called the Hansderma Skincool Ice Roller and I also use it to cool down my face after a run if it's a hot day and I'm running late and I need to stop sweating before I apply my tinted sunscreen.

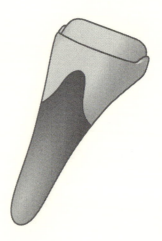

Swollen, Bloated and Puffy

The other roller I use is a jade roller. This handheld device has two jade rollers on either side of a jade handle. One side is a smooth roller that is small enough to use on my eyelids and the other 'acupuncture side' has rows of bumps that feel good when I roll them across my cheeks and the back of my neck. Sue Callison from Solidea Medical has a diagnosis of lymphedema after breast cancer and swears by the practice of rolling her face with a bumpy jade roller to improve her 'brain fog.' Check out more of her lymphedema rolling tips and tricks here: https://solideamedical.com/blogs/my-lymphedema-life-the-sue-callison-story

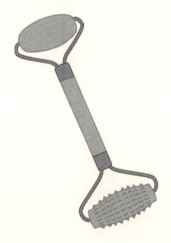

When face rolling, if you have swelling from head and neck cancer, please use a roller chilled to refrigerator temperature (not freezer) and use your self manual lymphatic drainage routine.

Beauty Masks

There are so many beauty masks out there, ranging from ultra-expensive ingredients to those $1 Korean masks at the H-Mart to homemade recipes with ingredients from your own kitchen. One hot ingredient right now when it comes to reducing inflammation is caffeine. Caffeine has a strong reputation for reducing swelling, but a study published in the July 2014 *International Wound Journal* found that caffeine may negatively affect wound healing (Ojeh et al, 2016). My advice: ask your plastic surgeon if you should use caffeine near your incision area before you try a face mask containing caffeine.

Raid your Freezer and Create Your Own Dunking Booth

Esthetician Renee Rouleau recommends a simple concoction to reduce puffiness – mix water, 15 ice cubes and ⅓ cup alcohol-free witch hazel in your sink and dunk your face 10 times. In a pinch, Rouleau also recommends taking a hot shower and allowing the water to massage your face, then grabbing anything in the freezer, even a frozen bag of peas or simple ice cubes to reduce under eye puffiness. Just hold against the eyes for five minutes to reduce swelling.

Information courtesy of www.ReneeRouleau.com, a website with helpful skin tips and advice from skin care expert and celebrity esthetician, Renée Rouleau.

Cold Spoons and Tea Bags

San Diego lifestyle blogger and author Lauryn Evarts has had to deal with facial swelling after having double jaw surgery as a teenager. She recommends using a spoon cooled in a glass of icewater for puffy eyes. She puts one side of the spoon on her eye area for two minutes or as long as she can stand it. She also wraps a teabag around a cold spoon and uses the spoon to hold the teabag against her eye area. Evarts is also a big fan of lymphatic drainage massage as well as using jade rollers and ice rollers. Find more tips from Evarts at her blog the Skinny Confidential

Swollen, Bloated and Puffy

here https://www.theskinnyconfidential.com/ and her Skinny Confidential Him & Her podcast here https://www.theskinnyconfidential.com/podcast/

Epsom Salt Bath

Massage therapists are famous for suggesting Epsom salt baths. We even gave out little baggies of Epsom salt to our clients at my massage school's student clinic. The Bone, Muscle and Joint team at the Cleveland Clinic recommends Epsom salts for reducing foot and ankle swelling. Their advice? "Soak your feet and ankles for 15 to 20 minutes in a cool bath filled with Epsom salt to relieve swelling-associated pain. If you have diabetic neuropathy in your feet, check the water with your hands first to avoid exposing your feet to extreme temperatures" (6 Best Fixes for Pain and Swelling in Your Feet and Ankles, 2016).

Hyperbaric Oxygen Therapy (HBOT) in a Pressurized Hyperbaric Chamber

Ingrid Marsten is a Certified Lymphedema Therapist in Los Angeles. I refer clients to her who have swelling after plastic surgery and are staying in the Los Angeles

/ Beverly Hills area. She recommends that clients with significant swelling look into whether Hyperbaric Oxygen Therapy (HBOT) would be an effective way to reduce swelling and improve wound healing. Ingrid stresses that the therapy should be in a pressurized chamber and her clients have found that at least three treatments are needed. Visit Ingrid Marsten's website http://ingridmarsten.abmp.com and contact her at ingridmarsten@gmail.com.

What Do Plastic Surgeons Use to Reduce Swelling?

Plastic Surgeon Gehaan D'Souza of Iconic Plastic Surgery in Carlsbad uses ice on procedures involving the eyelid and other areas with thin skin because ice causes blood vessels to contract. He gives Decadron intravenously during facelifts, rhinoplasties and neck lifts to decrease swelling and prescribes Medrol (an oral steroid) for patients with osteotomies and surgeries where the nasal bone is broken. D'Souza lets his patients use NSAIDs starting three days after surgery (use sooner and it will negatively affect the healing process) and use arnica after facelifts and rhinoplasty.

Follow Dr. D'Souza on Facebook here: https://www.facebook.com/IconicPlasticSurgery/

Dr. Kristina Tansavatdi is a fellowship-trained facial plastic and reconstructive surgeon in Westlake Village, CA. 'Dr. T' has several recommendations for her clients that reduce swelling after surgery, including drinking lots of water and decreasing salt intake. Recommended supplements include arnica to decrease bruising, bromelain to reduce swelling, turmeric to decrease inflammation and swelling as well as Vitamins A, C and Zinc for wound healing and antioxidants. Patients can also use ice, get up and move around as soon as possible after surgery, elevate the surgical site "to improve blood flow back to the heart and speed resolution of swelling" and get good sleep. Learn more about Dr. T at FacesbyDrT.com.

My favorite ways to reduce swelling:

_____

_____

_____

What to put in your face to reduce swelling

I wouldn't be a very good massage therapist if I didn't remind you to drink plenty of water! One of favorite massage therapist rituals is the one where we give our clients a glass of water after every massage. Remember: a pot of coffee or a 2 litre of soda is NOT a replacement for water. If you are swollen, trying to reduce your water intake will not reduce swelling. In some cases, a diuretic may help, but diuretics are not effective if your swelling is from lymphedema.

Please consult your physician before taking diuretic pills or 'natural' remedies or supplements. If you are swollen after an operation, be extra cautious. Supplements may also contain ingredients that thin the blood or have other harmful effects to those preparing for or recovering from surgery.

Here are five tips I follow that let me drink more water every day:

- A.M. – Drink 8-16 oz of water as soon as I wake up. We have our water in a copper jug next to the bed and drink first thing in the morning (drinking water stored in a copper vessel is a traditional Ayurvedic practice in parts of India). Sometimes we also like bottled sparkling water.

- Then I drink a cup of warm/hot liquid (tea or coffee) to get the digestive system working.

- Drink sips of warm water throughout the morning and have a cup of water an hour before lunch. I like to make an herbal tisane by adding a lemon slice, mint leaves or sliced ginger root to a cup of hot water.

- Afternoon: Consider adding berries or mint to your water to improve the taste. The ladies would drink Sassy Water at the office I used to work at before I switched careers. Sassy Water comes to us from the writers at Prevention Magazine and is a blend of lemons, ginger, mint and cucumbers (Sassy Water, 2011). For me, having an empty pitcher as my drinking goal for the end of the day helped me to keep track of my water intake. Find recipes for Sassy Water and other flavored waters here: http://www.prevention.com/food/cook/25-flat-belly-sassy-water-recipes.

Swollen, Bloated and Puffy

- Evening: Is your day so busy that you look up and it's 9 pm and you still haven't reached your daily water goal? Don't let this happen to you! Drink more often throughout the day. Experiment with your tolerance for liquids in the evening and don't let hydrating too late in the evening ruin your good night's sleep.

My ideas for drinking more water:

_____

_____

_____

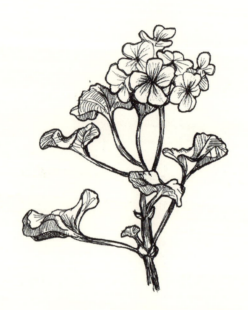

Geranium

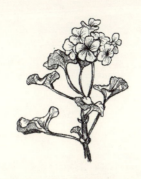

CHAPTER 3

WHAT TO WEAR TO REDUCE SWELLING

Many of my clients with lymphedema or plastic surgery have already had compression garments prescribed by their physician or certified lymphedema therapist. Compression garments are more than just a super expensive pair of shapewear. Their goal is not to smooth lumps and bumps, but to increase lymphatic flow by encouraging more fluid to re-enter the veins and enter the lymphatic system. Compression garments give our muscles something to press against when we move.

Compression garments can also work well to help non-lymphedema conditions, especially venous edema and varicose veins. There are three systems of veins in the leg, the superficial, perforator and deep. Factors that may lead to venous disorders include pregnancy, obesity, sedentary lifestyle, heredity (have your parents and relatives had venous issues? My grandma always wore support hose and I remember seeing her veins through her skin when I was a child), surgery or trauma, and my favorite – prolonged sitting or standing (pretty much every job out there). Remember that old wives tale that it's best to buy shoes at the end of the day, because your feet are bigger? They may be bigger because of swelling from sitting and standing all day.

Medical compression stockings sound really non-sexy but do a darn good job of reducing the end-of-day leg and foot swelling that comes with jobs with a lot of standing or sitting. A word about compression levels – 20 mmHg or more is the best level of compression of this type of swelling. Compression of less than 10 mmHg may still 'feel' tight and leave those lines on your calves after you wear them, but they are ineffective. If you have tried cheaper support stockings and not felt a difference in your legs, upgrade to a real pair of compression stockings with at least 20 mmHg. Do they cost more than socks at the department store? Yes, but if they work, it's worth it. Compression stockings may be covered under your Flexible Spending Account with a prescription, so if price is an issue, contact your doctor and ask if leg compression is right for you.

Over half of all women who have had two or more full-term pregnancies develop varicose veins and women who are pregnant are at increased risk of developing a blood clot. Compression socks and hosiery can help keep legs healthy. Simcox et al (2015) found that "pregnancy-associated pulmonary thromboembolism (VTE) remains a leading cause of direct maternal mortality in the developed world" (Simcox et al., 2015). Bottom line: If someone you love is pregnant, especially if she is dealing with swollen feet, get her compression socks instead of yet another newborn outfit.

Summer Swelling

Hot weather can increase swelling in our bodies because increased body heat can cause our blood vessels to expand. Some ladies cool their bandages or compression garments in the refrigerator for a while before wearing them. Experiment and see if a cooling ankle wrap (find them online or at the drugstore) helps with summer edema in the ankles and legs. If you have any medical issues with your legs or feet, check with your doctor first.

Look like an Olympian! Using Athletic Tape to Reduce Swelling

Remember the 2012 Olympics, when everyone had brightly colored tape on their bodies? The theory behind using athletic tape to reduce swelling is that the tape gently lifts the skin, changing the interstitial pressure and encouraging lymphatic vessels to take more fluid back to the heart. When the athletic tape is moved because of muscle contractions, the muscle pumping action also boosts lymphatic flow. Many physical therapists use athletic tape on their patients, particularly after joint replacements. Ask your Physical Therapist, Certified Lymphedema Therapist or Plastic Surgeon if using athletic tape to reduce swelling is right for you.

Kenzo Kase has an excellent guide for practitioners titled 'Kinesio Taping for Lymphoedema and Chronic Swelling.'

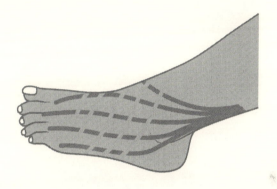

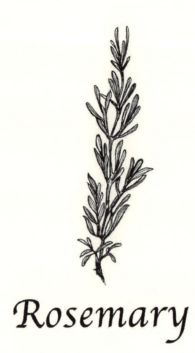

Rosemary

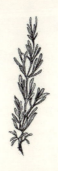

CHAPTER 4

LET'S USE GRAVITY AND OUR MUSCLES TO REDUCE SWELLING

How to use gravity while you sleep:

If you've had a facelift

I do love the RealSelf website. It's packed with plastic surgeons jumping to answer questions from ladies just like us! Many plastic surgeons on this site recommend sleeping with two pillows for a few weeks after facelift surgery. Elevating the head helps gravity drain the post-surgical swelling through the lymphatic system back to the heart. Find more tips at RealSelf.com and create a profile so you can start asking questions. My profile is at https://www.realself.com/user/3190163

If you've had surgery for breast cancer

The Memorial Sloan Kettering Cancer Center recommends that patients with a breast cancer diagnosis who can sleep on their side, sleep on the opposite side from their surgical site and rest their hand on 1-2 pillows placed in front of them. This will also help if you have shoulder pain. Use two pillows under your head. Place a third pillow lengthwise alongside your torso and a fourth pillow on top of your waist and hip so that one end of the top pillow rests on the pillow in front of you. This sounds like building a pillow fort, but it gives your arm better support as you sleep. Find more tips here: https://www.mskcc.org/cancer-care/patient-education/hand-and-arm-care-after-removal-axillary-lymph-nodes

Exercise to Reduce Swelling

Many of my tips on using exercise to reduce swelling come from my interactions with ladies with lymphedema. I am so grateful that they are so eager to support one another and share what has worked for them. When people with a lymphedema diagnosis exercise, they follow a few principles to increase their lymphatic flow.

Chapter 4: Let's Use Gravity and our Muscles to Reduce Swelling

The basics of lymphatic-boosting exercise include: mobilizing the joints of the body, wearing compression garments during exercise, utilizing the 'calf pump' by using the calves, and including slow, prolonged stretching.

The Bone, Muscle and Joint team at the Cleveland Clinic recommend exercises that move the ankle and knee joints like walking and swimming to reduce swelling (6 Best Fixes for Pain and Swelling in Your Feet and Ankles, 2016). The pressure of the water on the lower body when standing in a pool or other body of water is also effective for reducing swelling, so water aerobics is another great option. Don't have a pool in your backyard or a health club membership? See if you qualify for Silver Sneakers here: https://www.silversneakers.com/ There are over a dozen facilities with pools in San Diego that accept Silver Sneakers members.

Remember discovering the fun of bouncing on a trampoline when you were a kid? A gentler version of that exercise can help move lymph. Many lymphies (the sweet name people with a lymphedema diagnosis use to refer to themselves) gently bounce on a rebounder – a small trampoline with a safety bar / handrail. The movement of the ankle and knee joints and contraction and relaxation of the calf muscles help move lymphatic fluid out of the legs and feet. This may reduce swelling in your legs, ankles and feet. I have also heard of ladies using an under-the-desk elliptical machine at their desk to keep their ankle and knee joints moving while sitting for long periods at work.

I recommend the following stretches for improving lymphatic flow in the neck and face. Do several repetitions of each movement and take slow, deep belly breaths to activate your diaphragm as well.

Ear to Shoulder – In a seated position with relaxed shoulders, bend the head to the side, exhaling and stretching your neck so that your ear is as close to the shoulder as comfortable. Inhale and return head to an upright position and repeat on the other side.

Look to the Side – In a seated position with relaxed shoulders, inhale while turning the head to the side, being careful to keep the chin from tipping upward.

Exhale and turn the head all the way to the other side, then inhale to return the head to center.

Look Up and Down – In a seated position with relaxed shoulders, inhale while looking up toward the ceiling. Open the mouth a little to make the position more comfortable, then exhale and look down toward the ground. Inhale and return the head to center.

All of the lymphatic fluid in the face drains into the neck. Having proper lymphatic flow in the neck is essential for a healthy lymphatic system in the face, and these simple exercises done a few times a day can stimulate lymphatic flow in the neck.

Shoosh Lettick Crotzer has a complete full body 'lymphatic flow' gentle exercise video here: https://youtu.be/8btp39n5luc

Resie V. Collins is an Occupational Therapist and Certified Lymphedema Therapist here in San Diego. She recommends "muscle pumping" and abdominal breathing exercises to promote movement of the lymph.

If you need to add some variety to your workout, try using exercise bands instead of weights for joint moving exercises or perform your upper body workout while lying on a foam roller. The foam roller can support your head and spine, giving you a greater range of motion on the shoulder joint than when you are lying directly on the floor. If you are exercising after an operation, get permission from your doctor or physical therapist before trying any new exercises.

Physical Therapists Bob Schrupp and Brad Heineck along with Aaron Kast share a series of exercises for moving swelling out of the arms and legs on their YouTube account. Arm exercises include chicken wings, shoulder blade squeezes and deep breathing. Leg exercises include calf/ankle pumps with legs elevated, toe taps, butt squeezes and single knee to chest. Find these videos and more at https://www.youtube.com/user/physicaltherapyvideo and search for 'lymphedema.'

Chapter 4: Let's Use Gravity and our Muscles to Reduce Swelling

My favorite exercises that reduce swelling:

_____

_____

_____

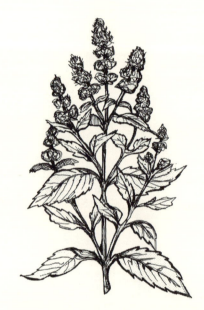

Peppermint

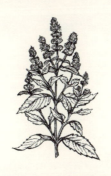

CHAPTER 5

HOW TO USE BREATHING TO BOOST YOUR LYMPHATIC SYSTEM

Deep diaphragmatic breathing can reduce swelling in the body by helping to move lymph. When's the last time someone taught you to breathe? 1. Swimming and 2. Childbirth, right?

We took our first breath seconds after birth and have been doing a pretty good job keeping ourselves alive ever since, so what's the big deal? The fact is, 83% of people with anxiety have breath dysfunction (Courtney, 2009). What does that mean? Too many of us take shallow breaths. Test yourself now by taking a breath with your hand placed over your belly button. Does your belly push out or does it remain motionless or get sucked in as you inhale? That's the difference between belly breathing and shallow breathing.

Try belly breathing by lying down on your back or in a reclining chair. Place your hands along the bottom of your ribcage, near your belly button. If you tend to get a tense jaw, try putting the tip of your tongue at the roof of your mouth to relax your jaw. Take a deep breath through your nose. Can you feel your rib cage widen and your tummy expand? Exhale completely. This is belly or diaphragmatic breathing. Belly breathing's worst enemies are the habit of holding our tummies in to look thinner and restrictive clothing that compresses our abdominal area. Consider wearing less restrictive clothing and letting your tummy move when breathing (but continue wearing doctor prescribed compression garments).

I have to confess, I feel conflicted when I teach about breathing. It feels wrong to waltz in with my white meditation teacher tunic and flowing pants fluttering in the ocean breeze and tell someone with a serious illness just to BREATHE and everything will be better.

Swollen, Bloated and Puffy

The reality: test it for yourself and see if it works for you. First, start noticing if you hold your breath to do everyday things, like standing, sitting, pulling a door or pushing something. It can be an unconscious habit. Then stop and add up all these moments of action. How many breaths are we skipping every day because we hold our breath every time we move? The solution is to time breathing so the pulling, pushing and lifting happens on an exhalation. We'll get the same momentum, and instead of holding our breath to brace our abdomen, practice the Knack (see Chapter 6).

I found out something fascinating about my body when I first began to meditate. I was plopped down on a meditation cushion in the second week of taking the mPEAK meditation program at the UC San Diego Center for Mindfulness. Our assignment was to focus on the breath, and suddenly I realized that I was expanding my lungs out in every direction when I breathed. I had always known to focus on my belly expanding outward to train myself to belly breathe while lying down. This new sensation felt more like an umbrella expanding, with the umbrella being my ribcage. I'm still shaking my head at myself that I never really paid attention to

Swollen, Bloated and Puffy

the way I breathed until I was 40 years old. Try belly breathing while seated and see if you can feel your ribcage expanding 360 degrees, too. Wrapping a scarf around your ribcage can help you feel the expansion.

If you want to get super advanced, research has found that alternate nostril breathing for 5 minutes each day helps heart function (Subramanian et al., 2016). To practice this type of breathing, close your left nostril with the left index finger and breathe in through the right nostril. Release the left nostril and close the right nostril with the right index finger and breath out through the left nostril. Breathe in through the left nostril and then release the right nostril. Breathe out through the right nostril. The idea is to breathe at a normal pace, exhaling and inhaling with one nostril, then exhaling and inhaling with the other nostril, alternating sides of the nose for five minutes.Some people use just one hand to close and release the nostrils. It's hard to explain without seeing it, so I suggest searching 'Nadi Shodhana' on YouTube.

Chapter 5: How to Use Breathing to Boost your Lymphatic System

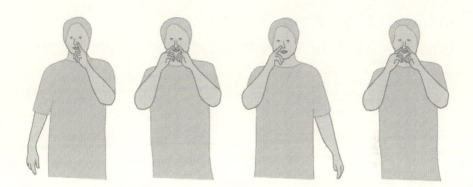

Every session of Manual Lymphatic Drainage I give to reduce swelling starts with encouraging the lymphatic system to move by using special massage strokes at the neck and the abdomen. There are some health benefits to beginning this way. The abdominal sequence includes massage of the abdomen toward the location of the cisterna chyli behind the navel, and then a series of deep belly breaths by the client. Belly breathing moves the diaphragm, which helps move the lymph up the thoracic duct and back into the bloodstream.

A fun way to stimulate lymphatic flow in the abdomen is blowing bubbles. One physical therapist I spoke to at a Lymphedema Seminar in Palm Springs in 2016 mentioned she recommends this 'therapy' to kids with primary lymphedema. Preparing to blow a string of bubbles is a natural way to breathe in deeply.

My favorite breath work exercises:

_____

_____

_____

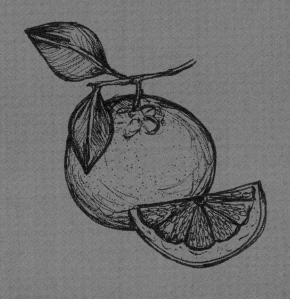

PART 3

LET'S HAVE A WOMAN TO WOMAN TALK ABOUT CONSTIPATION AND INCONTINENCE

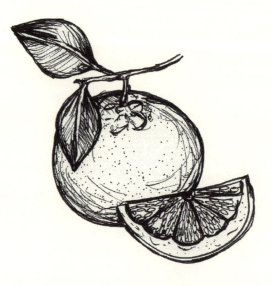

Grapefruit

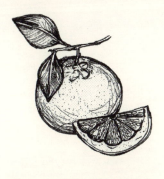

CHAPTER 6

BONUS CHAPTER FOR MOTHERS AND ALL LADIES OVER 40

Let me share what happens during so many of my lymphatic massage appointments. I am usually about five minutes into the massage, starting to work at the abdomen and I mention that this part of the treatment may change her bathroom habits in the next few days and not be worried about any temporary changes. Then my beautiful client who spends her life caring for others, sometimes before herself, opens up about her ongoing problems with constipation. If this sounds familiar, rest assured, you are not alone. One of my close friends suffers from constipation and has been to several doctors in search of relief and I myself have occasional incontinence and constipation. This is something that is not openly discussed in our society and as a result, many women are suffering in silence. It is my hope that these tips will help you and that you will lend this booklet to someone you love so they can help her, too. Being able to laugh and sneeze without worrying about leaking has improved my quality of life.

If I say pelvic floor muscle exercises, do you automatically think Kegels? Kegels get good PR, but when was the last time you did a full set of Kegels, and can you think of why you're doing them other than because it makes you better at sex? If you are a mother or over 40, you know you need to get serious about your pelvic floor. Don't let all those ads with ladies in linen pants walking along the beach convince you that incontinence is a normal part of aging.

We ask our pelvic floor to do some major supporting when we increase the pressure in our abdomen during the day. Times when the pelvic floor is under pressure include: lifting something, coughing, blowing our nose, sneezing, stepping down hard (AKA running), and for me especially, laughing so hard I cannot breathe.

Oh look, that list is also exactly when I can sometimes feel a little pee escape. Let's learn how to do the Knack

Swollen, Bloated and Puffy

and steady our pelvic floor so we can keep control over our bladders for as many years as possible. No one wants to have to wear adult diapers.

The Knack. The easiest way to practice is to do it when transferring from sitting to standing. Sit with your feet flat on the floor in front of you and your back straight. Breathe in and out. Now breathe in, tighten your anus (like you are drawing it up into your body, not trying to bear down) and lift your body to standing as you breathe out. The key is to tighten and draw in/up the pelvic floor muscles at the moment of exertion, whether that's coughing, laughing or lifting. When the activity is done, release your pelvic muscles.

Try using the Knack and see if it works for you. If it does, think about other ladies in your life that could benefit from learning it as well. Please share it with them. We do our best to hide incontinence issues from everyone, don't we? Lend your friends this booklet or invite them to join you at one of the meetings below.

Here in San Diego, Sharp and Scripps both offer classes on the pelvic floor. Find out more here:

Swollen, Bloated and Puffy

Sharp: Pelvic Health Community Talks https://www.sharp.com/health-classes/

Scripps: Learn How to Strengthen Your Pelvic Floor After Having a Baby https://www.scripps.org/health-and-wellness__events-and-classes

Not sure if you have a bladder issue? Take a Bladder Control Quiz here: https://www.voicesforpfd.org/assets/2/6/Bladder_Control_Quiz1.pdf

Constipation can make our tummy bloated and is a common problem after surgery. I recently met Michelle Lyons, an Irish physiotherapist, at the Klose Lymphedema Conference. She recommended several ways to improve digestion in her conference presentation and I will share some of her wisdom with you.

Her first tip is how to get your digestion started off on the right foot every morning. You will love this. She recommends a self-massage of the abdominal area to encourage that first poop of the day (see the diagram) and insists that we have our significant other or family member/friend get us a hot beverage to sip on while

Swollen, Bloated and Puffy

we are still in bed. Many people swear by coffee, but I prefer tea and am happy to report that my lovely husband does bring me Indian milk tea most every morning!

If you want to make your own essential oil blend for your morning abdominal massage, here's my home recipe. I add:

6 drops of sweet marjoram (Origanum majorana) essential oil

6 drops of rosemary (Rosmarinus officinalis) essential oil and

2 drops of black pepper (Piper nigrum) essential oil

to 15 ml of coconut oil

Mix well and store in a bottle in my night table.

You can also add a few drops of essential oil to your favorite stretch mark lotion/oil. I apply a little oil to my tummy and start right above my left hip bone, 'moonwalking' my fingertips in circles up to my ribcage, across my body and back down to my right hip. Ask your surgeon when it is OK to perform abdominal

Swollen, Bloated and Puffy

massage if you have had a recent abdominal surgery like a tummy tuck or a Cesarean section.

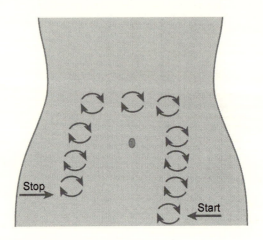

Constipation from anesthesia can be a distressing side effect of surgery. San Diego Naturopath Dr. Kristine Reese's treatment for post-surgical constipation includes hot water bottles or warm towels over the abdomen, massage, Super Aloe and/or Magnesium Citrate. She also recommends clients increase chewing, fiber and consumption of hot drinks. For more great wellness information, find Dr. Kristine Reese online at the Lotus Rain Facebook : https://www.facebook.com/LotusRainClinic/ the Lotus Rain Twitter: https://twitter.com/drreese and the LotusRain LinkedIn: https://www.linkedin.com/in/drkristinereese/

Swollen, Bloated and Puffy

Do you remember that medical mystery profiled in the NY Times 'Think Like a Doctor' column back in 2013? A 15-year-old nationally-ranked gymnast from Southern California suddenly had a swollen and distended belly, so huge that strangers thought she was pregnant, and she was forced to give up gymnastics. This story introduced me to the diagnosis of a 'functional gastrointestinal disorder,' which is basically when no test can figure out what is wrong with you because there is nothing abnormal about your body. Irritable bowel syndrome is an example of a 'functional gastrointestinal disorder.' It turns out one of the reasons this teenaged girl became so constipated and bloated was because she had a pelvic floor dysfunction (Sanders, 2013). She needed to learn how to poop correctly.

When is the last time anyone taught you to poop? If the answer was decades ago or never, today is your lucky day! When you are going to poop, Michelle Lyons recommends using a product like the Squatty Potty or a child's stepping stool to bring the knees up and make passing a bowel movement easier. I first discovered how much easier it is to poop while squatting when I visited my husband's parents in Trivandrum, Kerala

Swollen, Bloated and Puffy

(India). They had a western-style toilet in the house, but I soon encountered the infamous Turkish toilet in restaurants. I had to straddle a hole in the ground and found that squatting deeply was easier than trying to 'hover.' My bowel movements were easier from this deep squatting position. I have a toilet stool in my bathroom now and find that it pretty much replicates that ideal squatting angle.

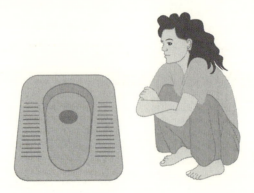

You have a toilet stool and you know the proper pooping position, the next step is to make sure you're not inadvertently squeezing when you think you're pushing. Michelle Lyons taught us the fun shortcut to trying to figure out pooping – just relax your pelvic floor and let nature take it's course. How? By making your pooping zen sound.

Swollen, Bloated and Puffy

How can I find my own personal pooping zen sound, Kathleen?

Sit comfortably and focus on your pelvic floor. Now breathe in and make one of the following sounds: a Monster roar, a Librarian's Shhhhh, a snake's hisss, a cow's moo, or blowing through an imaginary straw. Let each exhale be a different sound on the list and feel which sound is the best at relaxing your anus and pelvic floor. For me, it's the cow's moo.

Fast forward to your next poop. You're on the toilet, sitting with feet on your footstool and you feel the urge. Inhale and exhale normally, making your sound with each exhale. The sound will let you 1. Not hold your breath or strain, 2. Relax your pelvic floor and 3. May alarm the dog. Yes, it feels embarrassing the first few times, but it's worth it if you can become more regular.

You might also try relaxing the abdominal muscles and giving yourself a lower back massage while on the toilet. Focus on gently massaging the skin around your tailbone in an upward direction.

If you continue to have issues with going to the bathroom or pelvic pain, there is help! Your doctor

Swollen, Bloated and Puffy

can refer you to an in-network physical therapist with expertise in the pelvic floor. You can find a complete list of practitioners across the country here: https://hermanwallace.com/practitioner-directory

Michelle Lyons also wants you to make friends with your pelvic floor (and YES, it means you have to touch your anus).

Michelle recommends the following: "Comfortably position yourself, ideally lying on your side with your knees bent. You should be wearing leggings/yoga pants or just your underwear. Reach back and place one finger gently over your anus, now move it to the side, still quite close to the anus. Take a deep breath in, exhale and relax all your muscles, especially your pelvic floor muscles. Take another breath in; this time as you exhale, imagine you are closing the opening to your anus then lifting up and in. Count to 5 out loud (just to make sure you are not holding your breath!). Then on your next exhale, relax all the muscles around your anus and breathe normally. Now try this without having your finger reach back. Can you feel the muscles close your anus & lift up and in? Can you feel

Swollen, Bloated and Puffy

them relax again? Can you do this while sitting and while standing? Congratulations! You have effectively located, contracted & relaxed your pelvic floor."

Check out Michelle Lyon's website at CelebrateMuliebrity.com and find more information on constipation here: https://www.voicesforpfd.org/assets/2/6/Constipation.pdf

Food sensitivities are becoming more recognized as a possible source of abdominal bloating and other digestive symptoms. I have heard wonderful stories of women whose digestion improved radically after investing in a food sensitivity test and faithfully following a modified diet. Naturopathic Doctors are a good resource for finding out more about this treatment.

I have been eating yogurt with live active cultures for years, but the first time I had a doctor actually recommend probiotics to me was here in San Diego before my recent trip to India. I digested the spicy foreign food much better than I had during previous trips to visit my in-laws (my husband is from India) so I did some research online to find out whether probiotics

Swollen, Bloated and Puffy

could be useful in recovering from plastic or cosmetic surgery procedures like facelifts or tummy tucks.

I had heard the common sense explanation that 'antibiotics destroy intestinal bacteria and probiotics help repopulate your gut flora,' but surprisingly, it was hard for me to find solid scientific evidence for adding probiotics to a post-surgery diet. I found one study that is targeted to trauma nurses taking care of patients in the hospital. In the January 2017 Journal of Trauma Nursing article 'Probiotics for Trauma Patients: Should We Be Taking a Precautionary Approach?' Heather A. Vitko provides a balanced overview of the use of probiotics in hospitals. Research has found that probiotics decrease rates of infection and antibiotic-associated diarrhea, but Vitko cautions that probiotics are only regulated as supplements. According to Vitko, the most common probiotics used in research are Lactobacillus and Saccharomyces boulardii (Vitko et al, 2017).

My favorite ways to reduce abdominal bloating:

_____

_____

_____

Have You Heard Of This??? Crazy Ways to Increase the Flow

- Take your swelling for a ride: Some lymphies have found that using their riding lawnmower, going for a ride on a motorcycle or sitting in a vibrating chair has reduced their lymphedema.

- Some clients with lymphedema after Head and Neck Cancer have found that using a paint roller can reduce swelling in the back of the neck and upper back. Try this by rolling a new, clean, dry paint roller from the neck and spine downward and outward to direct fluids to lymph nodes in the armpit.

Why Am I Swollen There?

- If you have hemorrhoids: top Cleveland Clinic 'doctor-approved' home remedies include a sitz bath, soaking a cotton pad in witch hazel, pure aloe and Epsom salts/glycerin compress (7 Best and Worst Home Remedies for Your Hemorrhoids, 2016).

- If you have arthritis swelling: unlike lymphedema, arthritis swelling is often in the synovial fluid of the joint. According to the Arthritis Foundation, symptoms can be reduced by applying heat or cold to the area, whichever brings more relief. Natural remedies include heating pads, warm showers, heated pool or ice packs. Only apply heat/cold for under 20 minutes at a time and let the skin return to a normal temperature before applying again (Freeman, n.d.) Physical Therapist and Certified Lymphedema Therapist Linda Roherty recommends dipping arthritic joints in paraffin wax as a heat treatment because the paraffin molds more closely to finger and toe joints. Paraffin bath machines like the one I use can be found online for under $50, and the wax can be remelted and used again by the same person.

- It might be Cushing's Syndrome: According to the Mayo Clinic, "Too much cortisol can produce some of the hallmark signs of Cushing syndrome — a fatty hump between your shoulders, a rounded face, and pink or purple stretch marks on your skin" (Cushing Syndrome, n.d.). If you have these signs, mention them to your doctor.

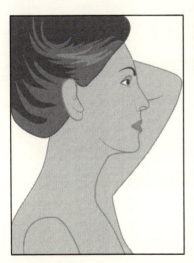 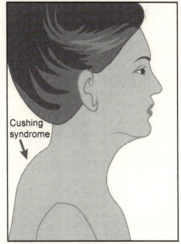

- What about Lipedema and Dercum's Disease: these fat disorders are not well known and many people are left undiagnosed or misdiagnosed for years. Find out more about symptoms and

Swollen, Bloated and Puffy

treatment at the Fat Disorders Research Society http://www.fatdisorders.org/. Dr. Karen Herbst, Director of the University of Arizona TREAT (Treatment, Research and Education of Adipose Tissue) program, offers a list of medicine and supplements for those with Lipedema and Dercum's disease. This list could be a great way to jumpstart a conversation on supplementation between you and your doctor. You can find her list here: http://treat.medicine.arizona.edu/sites/treat.medicine.arizona.edu/files/medicine-and-supplements-handout-fdrs-2016_without_color.pdf

- There are some forms of swelling that manual lymphatic drainage cannot help. If only one leg is swollen and the swelling came on suddenly, let your doctor know immediately, it may be a blood clot. If a limb is swollen because of infection, a blood clot, heart failure or kidney failure, MLD is contraindicated and I recommend you seek the care of a doctor.

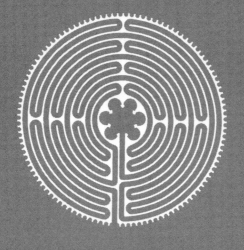

PART 4

YOUR IMMUNE SYSTEM

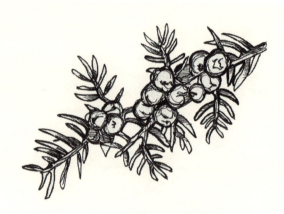

Juniper

7 WORRIED SICK - HOW TO IMPROVE YOUR IMMUNE SYSTEM

Many people are interested in lymphatic massage as a way to detox or improve their immune system. In addition to manual lymphatic drainage, practices like meditation, getting enough sleep, proper exercise, dry brushing, massage, music, positive emotions, laughter and friendship can also positively affect our immune system function. In fact, Integrative Cardiologist Dr. Mimi Guarneri states in her book *108 Pearls to Awaken Your Healing Potential* that "stress is our immune system's nemesis. Not only do we get sick more easily under stress, we find it more difficult to recover" (Guarneri, 2017). Read on for tips on how to add these practices to your life.

How Can I Try Meditation?

Let's meditate together for a few minutes and then I'll share some tips I learned the hard way in my first few years of meditating. If you have tried to meditate before but were frustrated because you had too many thoughts or couldn't sit still, please give it another try!

Sit comfortably. No, you don't have to twist yourself into lotus position or change into an all white outfit. Sit on a chair with your feet on the floor, if that's easiest. I'm short, so I sit on the couch and cross my legs. Many meditators find it more comfortable when their hips are above their knees, so they sit on a meditation cushion or a yoga block. Place your hands comfortably in your lap, or, if you want to get fancy, place your hands on your knees and try one of the hand mudras pictured in this chapter. Settle in and get a sense of allowing the chair to hold you. Close your eyes or keep them open and gaze down the front of your nose to the floor. Connect with your breathing and find a place where you feel the sensation of breathing the strongest. It may be at the tip of the nose, where we can feel the cool air entering and warmer air leaving our body. It may be in the belly. Gently focus on that area and breathe naturally for ten breaths. If a thought comes, gently let it go and refocus on your breath. After ten breaths, wiggle your fingers and toes and open your eyes if they are closed. Give yourself a minute to return to reality. You did it!

Yes, I am a certified Meditation Teacher and taught Meditation and Mindfulness at IPSB College in San

Diego, but I didn't always meditate. I began practicing meditation during a period of high anxiety in my life. I had just sprained my ankle, forcing me to cancel running a half marathon race for which I had been training over the previous three months. I had moved cross-country that past summer for my husband's job, which meant a career change, and I was due to start massage school in a few weeks.

As I sat on the meditation cushion those first few times, I heard all my anxieties surfacing in the quiet of my mind. My sarcastic New Yorker inner voice reminded me that if I wanted to sit around and be reminded of how disappointed and scared I was, I could do it with a glass of wine instead of paying hundreds of dollars to a meditation instructor. But I didn't quit. Soon I became more experienced at meditation. I was able to recognize those anxious thoughts and let go of them before they turned into full-blown stories.

Those first few times, I was feeling the effects of a major meditation misconception — that meditation is going to be like a day at the beach — just relaxing, not thinking, every care magically whisked away.

Swollen, Bloated and Puffy

The reality is that meditation for beginners will always involve thoughts, and often exactly the thoughts we don't want to think about. Meditation reduces anxiety not by ending anxious thoughts but by allowing them to pass – like a child learning to play catch with a ball.

Have you ever seen major league baseball triple play? Let's agree to not talk about the Padres, it's a rebuilding year. The ball is in and out of the glove in record time because the players saw the ball coming and were able to recognize it and then let it leave their glove. If anxious thoughts are like a baseball, the goal of learning to work with the ball effectively is to not hold onto the ball.

OK, so we'll get the ball out of our proverbial glove, you say. But first, let's consider another major meditation misconception. This one is about the best way to let a thought pass. Many beginning meditators believe that thoughts during meditation mean they are a failure and that 'forcing' themselves not to think and berating themselves when they do is the only way to 'win' at meditating. I'm type A, goal oriented, driven. I get it.

Swollen, Bloated and Puffy

Instead, we can let thoughts pass by recognizing and naming them ("thinking" or "this is anxiety") and returning to the breath. Name, return. Name, return. Name, return. Much like a player catches hundreds of balls during a baseball drill, this process can happen hundreds of times during meditation and it is an essential skill to develop. The magic part for me is when the skill of recognizing a thought starts appearing in my everyday life. Instead of getting caught up in anxious thoughts, I can begin to recognize them when the first thought comes to mind and I'm able to label it before it overwhelms me.

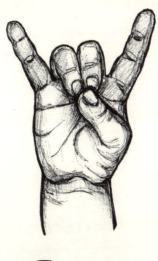

Apana

Swollen, Bloated and Puffy

This 'meditation thing' worked for me and I became so impressed by the positive effects of meditation in my life I trained in Sedona with former Chopra Center Program Director and and best-selling author Sarah McLean to become a meditation teacher. As I mentioned before, I taught the meditation & mindfulness class at IPSB in San Diego. On the first night of class, we discussed tips for how to fit a regular meditation practice into a busy schedule. Here's what I shared with them about how new meditators can make our practice into a daily habit.

Tip 1 – Choose Your Space

The first tip is to select one spot in the house or yard to meditate and keep necessary items nearby – pillows, blankets, gratitude journal etc. Meditating at the ocean or a canyon? Place all needed items in a bag and give the bag a 'home.'

Tip 2 – Choose Your Meditation

The second is to determine in advance how long and which meditation will be used. A meditation app like Insight Timer can provide support for silent and guided meditations. Important — learn a lesson from me and don't shock yourself out of the meditation with a loud, annoying alarm. I have to admit, I used to use the alarm on the stove before I found Insight Timer. Make sure the sound is soothing. In a pinch, use a relaxing song from your phone's music collection as the alarm.

Tip 3 – Choose Your 'Reminder'

The third is to pick a 'reminder' for our meditation, an event that happens right before it's time to meditate. That could be walking the dog, making a cup of tea, or returning from driving the kids to school. The 'reminder' will remind us it is time to meditate and the location, supplies, time and type of meditation are already decided. All that's left to do is enter into the present moment.

My Space, Meditation and 'Reminder':

_____
_____
_____

Swollen, Bloated and Puffy

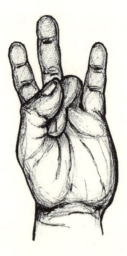

Surya

Once we have a regular meditation schedule, we might want to fit tiny meditative moments into the rest of our day. Here are five ways we can relax, no matter how busy our schedule is.

If we have five minutes — try a body scan. Sitting or lying down, find a comfortable position and gently focus on different parts of our body in this relaxing technique. Start by feeling our toes for two breaths, then feel each different body part, switching every second inhale. Breathe and feel the feet, ankles, lower legs and knees. Continue to focus on how our body feels from

Swollen, Bloated and Puffy

the inside of your thighs, hips, lower back, abdomen, upper back, shoulders, chest, arms, hands and fingers. We can finish our body scan by feeling inside our neck, jaw, face, ears and scalp, each for two breaths. Finally, focus on our entire body breathing peacefully for a few breaths. This can be done first thing in the morning or at night in bed or when we are a passenger in a car.

If we can spare two minutes twice a day, try the 4-7-8 breathing technique. Inhale deeply for four counts, hold our breath for seven counts, and exhale for eight counts with a sigh, then repeat for four cycles. The exercise gives us a minute to pause and regroup, as well as turn off our body's fight or flight response so we feel less stressed.

If we have one minute – focus on our breath. This exercise can be done at our desk or even in a tense meeting! Take a slow deep inhale through our nose, then exhale through our nose. Count to two, then inhale again. Pausing in between breaths brings relaxation.

If we are waiting in line – whether at the grocery store or for our morning coffee, take 30 seconds to notice what is going on in the body. With each breath, focus

Swollen, Bloated and Puffy

on relaxing the muscles around the eyes, then the forehead, then the jaw, then letting the shoulders be at ease.

Where do we feel tense in our body? Often, it's not just where we think. Try this trick – imagine you are making a business presentation and were just asked a question you can't answer. Feel that anxiety in your body. Now, notice what parts of your body tensed up. Your hands? Your face? Your belly? Focus on relaxing your personal list of tense body parts the next time you need a dose of relaxation. For me, it's in my chest and, weirdly, my hamstrings.

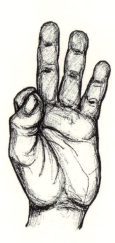

Vayu

Swollen, Bloated and Puffy

Tell me more about Guided Meditation

Guided meditation is a great resource for new and experienced meditators who would like more support for our meditation practice. In this type of meditation, a meditation teacher verbally guides us, offering prompts and letting us know when the meditation is completed. Apps like Insight Timer offer a variety of guided meditations. A great option for jumpstarting a meditation practice is to take a 'meditation challenge.' A meditation challenge is a program where a meditation teacher will choose a meditation each day for us to follow for a period of time. Try Refinery 29's 30 Day Meditation Challenge here: http://www.refinery29.com/2016/08/118362/meditation-30-day-challenge

One final tip: There are dozens of different types of meditation and you don't have to like every one. If you find one you dislike intensely, finish out the meditation session and then try a different one in your next meditation session. For me, it was a mantra meditation that really annoyed me. Give yourself a few weeks or months of meditating, then playfully and curiously try the disliked meditation again. If it's still annoying, just switch back the next day to something you like more. But maybe like me, you'll find that you end up liking it better the second time you try it.

How Can I Get More Sleep?

Do you need more sleep? If the answer isn't an instant YES, take a simple test by answering the five questions of the S.A.T.E.D. assessment:

- Satisfaction: Are you satisfied with your sleep?
- Alertness: Can you stay awake all day without getting sleepy?
- Timing: Are you asleep (or trying) between 2:00 and 4:00 a.m.?
- Efficiency: Does it take you less than 30 minutes to fall asleep?
- Duration: Do you sleep between 6 – 8 hours every night?

Why Is Sleep Important?

I can feel the negative effects of a poor night's sleep the next day. Does this happen to you, too? Too little sleep is not only annoying, but it's also bad for our bodies in several ways.

According to the National Institutes of Health, the brain's glymphatic system (nope, that's not a misspelling, it's so named because it is regulated by glial cells) filters beta-amyloid from the cerebrospinal fluid more effectively when we sleep. Literally, sleep lets our brain clean itself better because brain cells take up less space in our head when we are sleeping (How sleep clears the brain, 2013).

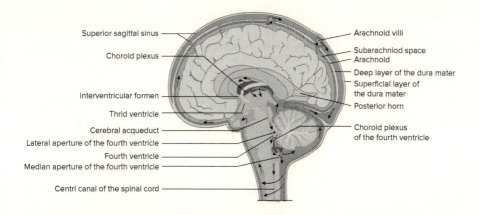

An Emory University study surveyed over 500 middle-aged men and women and found that those who slept six hours or less at night had higher levels of three "inflammatory markers" including "fibrinogen, IL-6 and

Swollen, Bloated and Puffy

C-reactive protein" compared to participants who slept over six hours each night. (Poor Sleep Quality Increases Inflammation, 2010).

As a meditation teacher, I know that our number one way to detoxify from the stress of the day is through a good night's sleep. Meditation can also release stress, but sleep is key to robust health. If you want to take a deep dive into all the ways that a solid eight hours of sleep positively affects your life, pick up a copy of *Why We Sleep* by Matthew Walker, a professor of Neuroscience and Psychology at the University of California, Berkeley, and Director of the University's Sleep and Neuroimaging Laboratory.

Does your room have blackout curtains, a humidifier and the finest bed linens on a comfortable mattress and yet you still can't get to sleep at night? The answer may be in your pre-bedtime rituals. A Detroit-based study of sleep hygiene among insomniacs found that drinking alcohol, smoking near bedtime and taking naps during the day were common practices in those with insomnia (Jefferson et al, 2005). This is an excellent example of what NOT to do! My biggest

Swollen, Bloated and Puffy

battle is limiting contact with electronics within a half hour of my bedtime. Looking at just one more website or Facebook update is simply too attractive to me and I can easily stay up an hour past my bedtime and then spend another half hour lying in bed with thoughts spinning in my mind. A better bedtime ritual? Set an alarm on my phone for a half hour before bedtime and spend that time reading or performing my pre-sleep essentials — brushing my teeth and applying lotion to my face and body. Maybe spending time with loved ones or petting my dog? Gazing at the stars or the moon, which are beautiful in San Diego when we don't have a marine layer. Reviewing the needs of the next day and making sure I have prepared everything so I am not stressed or rushed in the morning. Making notes of everything left to do so I won't have to try to remember them right before I fall asleep.

My Dozen Tips for Falling Asleep

- I avoid napping late in the afternoon or evening — allowing myself to get increasingly sleepy

Swollen, Bloated and Puffy

- I don't drink alcohol in the later afternoon or evening or eat heavy foods too close to bedtime – it ruins my sleep
- We don't have television or other distracting electronics in the bedroom (this is one we are still working on)
- I don't use my bed for lounging – I train my body to associate the bed only with sleep
- I don't use LED light within an hour of bedtime – I allow my body to sense it is night time. We have a sleep light bulb in the lamp at the bedside table and I have sleep glasses that block out blue light
- I give myself a 9 hour window for sleep at night – I try to wake up without an alarm and don't use a snooze button
- I get into a habit of going to bed and waking up at the same time each day, even weekends
- We don't have clocks within view of the bed
- I set an alarm 30 minutes before bedtime so I can start my bedtime rituals

Swollen, Bloated and Puffy

- I like using a warm foot bath to relax. After removing my feet from the foot bath, the drop in body temperature allows me to fall asleep more quickly
- We leave the screen door to our balcony open at night. Alternately, we could also turn the thermostat down to 65 degrees. Back East, we called it 'sleeping weather' when we left the window open at night in cooler spring and fall days
- I use a meditation or breathing techniques if thoughts are preventing sleep

Still tossing and turning? Try these types of guided meditation for sleep:

- Mantra Meditation – Repeat a word or phrase silently over and over. The repetition can be very soothing and relaxing, but some people find that mantras can be energizing, so try it and see for yourself
- Body Scan – focus on and relax parts of the body from the head to the feet

- Yoga Nidra – This type of yoga doesn't involve movement at all! Instead, the meditator will enter a deep 'yogic' sleep

The National Institutes of Health offers a free online Guide to Healthy Sleep here: https://www.nhlbi.nih.gov/files/docs/public/sleep/healthy_sleep.pdf

How to Exercise to Balance the Immune System

As an RRCA-Certified Running Coach, I am intrigued by the relationship between exercise and our immune system. Research has shown that moderate exercise helps the immune system but efforts like intense training and racing can depress immune function in mice (Reynolds, 2009). When athletes train hard, we have also to incorporate immune-boosting and stress-busting practices in our schedules. For me, that is a healthy diet, meditation, enough sleep, massages and no alcohol (find out more about how alcohol affects the immune system here: https://pubs.niaaa.nih.gov/publications/Hangovers/beyondHangovers.pdf).

While many of my non-athletic colleagues focus only on the advice that too much training has a negative effect on the immune system, I am much more interested in the fact that adding moderate amounts of exercise to one's lifestyle will balance the immune system!

Looking for gentler exercise? Research has found that participating in Tai Chi or Qi Gong can improve the immune system (Rogers, 2009). Find free Tai Chi and Qi Gong classes in San Diego here: http://www.sdce.edu/schedule#/emeritus

Good news for patients with a cancer diagnosis – research has also found that exercise can improve chemo brain (Phillips et al 2016) which is difficulty with retrospective and prospective memory. Prescription antidepressants may affect the effectiveness of systemic cancer therapies, so a natural approach could be a good alternative.

Dry Brushing

Dry brushing is the ritual of brushing the skin with a specific type of brush in order to improve the skin and engage the lymphatic system. But does it work

Swollen, Bloated and Puffy

and what are some tips to have the best results? I first encountered dry brushing in massage school. We were told to buy dry brushes and practice dry brushing daily for a week. I saw improvement in the softness of my skin. Now that I have advanced training in manual lymphatic drainage, I am interested in the benefits of dry brushing for both the skin and lymph drainage. The trouble is that most of what I read online are the exact same 'rules' with no explanation of where they came from or if they have any backing in science.

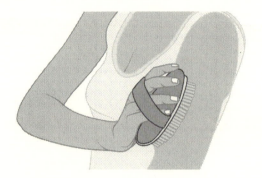

Let's tackle the science part first. I found three articles that consult medical experts. The Cleveland Clinic recommends dry brushing to promote lymph flow and drainage (Starkey, 2015). The New York Times reports Dr. Tina S. Alster, a clinical professor of dermatology at Georgetown University Medical Center finds that dry brushing helps the lymphatic system "work better" (Saint Louis, 2010). The University of Maryland Medical Center includes dry brushing on its extensive list of ways to reduce fluid retention (Ehrlich, 2016).

It looks like there is some basis for trying it. Now, what about the 'rules'? First, the rule about always brushing toward the heart is simplistic and works for the most part, but isn't as effective as brushing in the direction of lymphatic flow. If you have secondary lymphedema, dry brushing can be a good idea and has worked for other lymphies, but direct the fluid to working lymph nodes just like you do in self-MLD. My keys to dry brushing are using a brush that is soft and caring for the integrity of our skin, especially if our immune system is compromised. The stroke should not just pet or glide across the skin. We have to move the skin in order to open up the lymph capillaries and reduce swelling. Tip – some ladies with lymphedema have found that they remove a LOT of dead skin the first time they dry brush, so lay on a towel or dry brush outside if this could be a concern for you.

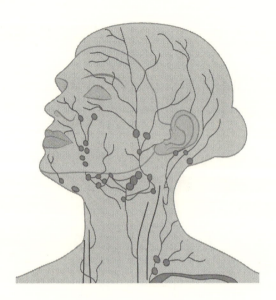

My Top Tips on how to Dry Brush:

- If you use natural bristles, make sure your dry brush has never been used (gotten wet) in the shower or bath. Keep a separate one just for brushing

- If you are cautious of using natural bristles because of the potential for skin damage, some lymphies use manmade bristles and even a pet hair brush for dry brushing

- Brush in strokes that follow the pathway of the lymphatic system

Swollen, Bloated and Puffy

- Dry brush before shower or exercise, when skin is dry
- Don't brush too much! Stop before skin becomes sensitive or turns red
- Moisturize after you dry brush (or after the post-brushing shower)

If you want to try dry brushing and have a normally functioning lymphatic system, use the following diagram:

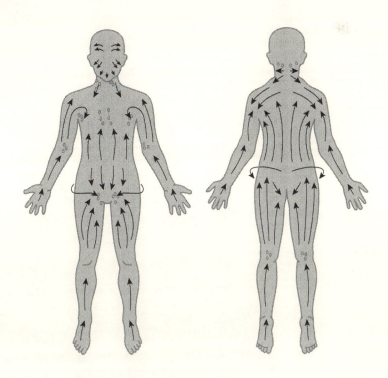

Swollen, Bloated and Puffy

If you have had orthopedic, reconstructive or plastic surgery (with no lymph nodes biopsied or removed) a few weeks ago and have swelling near your incision scar, which likely means that the lymphatics are impaired. Don't worry, they are busy healing, but can't work at 100% just yet. Ask your surgeon for an OK before trying dry brushing, and avoid brushing over the scar, as it is busy healing, too. You can often brush all other areas of your body, only avoiding the skin around the surgical area.

A fellow massage therapist mentioned to me that he enjoys 'multitasking' and does his 10 minutes of oil pulling while he dry brushes his body. Oil pulling is an ancient Ayurvedic practice thought to boost the immune system by removing bacteria from the mouth. It's basically swishing either a tablespoon of coconut or sesame oil (not toasted) in the mouth and 'pulling' it through your teeth for 10 – 20 minutes and then spitting the liquid into the trash. Shanbhag, V. K. L. (2017) put together an informative review of scientific literature on the practice. I have listed a link to 'Oil pulling for maintaining oral hygiene – A review' in the bibliography (Shanbhag, 2017).

Swollen, Bloated and Puffy

Massage

Everyone knows that Swedish and Deep Tissue massage is relaxing, that's why it's the go-to gift for Mother's Day. But isn't it just an expensive, pamper-me type experience? The American College of Physicians released an evidence-based clinical practice guideline in *Annals of Internal Medicine* stating that physicians and patients should treat acute or subacute low back pain with non-drug therapies such as superficial heat, massage, acupuncture, or spinal manipulation (Quaseem, 2017). Massage has also been proven as a very relaxing way to reduce insomnia and boost the immune system (Adults Demonstrate Modified Immune Response After Receiving Massage, 2010).

If you have reduced range of motion or increased sensitivity around your surgery scars, incorporating 10 minutes of scar massage into your regular hour long massage sessions can bring relief. Scar massage techniques can be used by a trained massage therapist starting two months after your surgery. I have advanced training in post breast surgery scar massage and have worked with orthopedic scars as well. I recommend starting with three weekly one hour full body massage sessions including scar massage and mobilization and then reassessing your pain levels and range of motion before creating a long term care plan.

Once you have your doctor's permission to start massaging your surgery area, here are my tips for self-massage on scars:

- Let scars heal for two months before starting self massage
- Use a small amount of Sesame or Mahanarayan oil (spot test to make sure you are not allergic)
- Use light pressure, move slowly and stop if skin becomes red or little red dots form on the skin
- Use the strokes I demonstrated to you after your first massage
- Focus on moving the scar and skin horizontally instead of pushing down
- Limit self-massage on scars to less than 5 minutes a day

Convinced that massage can help you reduce anxiety and muscle tension? My top tip will be to schedule a relaxing massage with me, but I'll also share some tips on how to massage your significant other, how to make a 'home spa' evening and how to use reflexology to reduce swelling.

Couples can increase intimacy levels through regular giving and receiving of touch. My husband Arun loves to hike and rock climb, and he is pretty lucky that he's married to a massage therapist! Here's what I have found works for him. A welcome massage in the morning might be light friction, using the whole hand over large areas like the back or front of legs. Mimic the pressure you use to warm your hands when you rub them together on a very cold day. This will get the blood flowing and prepare the body for activity.

After a busy day at work or if a partner is still on his/her computer and is willing to accept touch, try a simple shoulder massage. The neck and shoulder muscles love attention. Focus on the back of the shoulders and neck and practice on yourself first to get the correct pressure (if your loved on is a cancer survivor, use lighter pressure and slower strokes). After placing a little lotion in your palm, make a duck's bill with your

Swollen, Bloated and Puffy

hand, like you are playing with a sock puppet, and place your hand on your opposite shoulder. Rub the area, focusing on bringing the trapezius muscle up, then switch to the back of the neck, gently pushing the neck muscles toward the spine.

A great massage idea for the end of the day is a foot rub. Pregnant women and people on their feet all day love this massage. Apply lotion to the feet and rub gently at first, asking him or her to let you know what feels best. For an extra treat, fill a dishpan with warm water and let the one you love soak their feet for 5 minutes before the massage!

Speaking of soaking the feet, try my 'home spa' idea the next time you have sore feet. Yes, setting up a fancy home spa can cost hundreds of dollars. Instead, try a 'weeknight spa' that's simple and easy, using many items you already have in your home.

Your shopping list: A bag of Epsom salts from the drug store and your favorite soothing essential oil. Lavender (Lavandula angustifolia) and geranium (Pelargonium graveolens) are good choices.

Swollen, Bloated and Puffy

First, take off your work clothes and wrap yourself up in your favorite robe. Start with a dishpan from the kitchen, body lotion and a few washcloths from your closet. Mix a small handful of Epsom salts and one or two drops of your essential oil into the bottom of the dishpan. Place the dishpan in front of your couch and fill it with really warm water, letting the salt dissolve while you wet the washcloths at your sink and wring them out before microwaving them for 30 seconds or until steamy. My shortcut is to fill my tea kettle to the top, boil the water and use some for the foot bath, mixing with cooler water, some for the washcloths and the rest for a cup of Echinacea tea. Grab your tea, the hot washcloths and your lotion and head over to your foot bath. Sit down and place your feet in the foot bath. Unroll the washcloth and press it into your face. Aaahhh HEAVEN! You can rub additional washcloths on your arms, legs and the back of the neck. Let the stress of the day drain away. After the foot bath has gone cold, give yourself a foot, neck and shoulder massage with your lotion.

Have you heard of Reflexology for improving lymphatic function? Some reflexologists target certain areas of

Swollen, Bloated and Puffy

the foot during a foot massage to improve lymphatic function. Does it work? Who knows. The areas include the big toe and the little toe for the neck lymph nodes, the top of the foot near the toes for the chest, breast and back lymphatics, the side of the foot right behind where the little toe begins for the armpit lymph nodes, and the crease on the top of the foot where the ankle begins for the inguinal lymph nodes. If you enjoy reflexology foot massage, and want to learn more, *Therapeutic Reflexology* by Paula S. Stone is a good resource.

Music can 'harmonize' the immune system

Board Certified neurologic music therapist Angela Neve from the San Diego-based Music Therapy Center of California shared with me that music therapy can "improve your mood by producing endorphins to help you feel good, boost your immune system by increasing cancer-killing cells, which can help the body combat cancer as well as other viruses, including AIDS" and "reduce anxiety" by decreasing cortisol. Neve's tip is to practice deep breathing and relaxation techniques while listening to slow tempo, wordless music. Once we have taught our body that listening to the musical piece is a signal to relax, we can play it when we are anxious or cannot sleep as a way to help us move into relaxation. Find out more about music therapy at TheMusicTherapyCenter.com and visit their Facebook page at Facebook: https://www.facebook.com/themusictherapycenter

Scientists reviewed 400 research papers and found that listening to music had major health benefits when it came to managing our mood, stress and immunity. Let's focus specifically on immunity. Listening to music prompts our body to increase production of both immunoglobulin A (an antibody) and natural killer cells (Chanda & Levitin, 2013). I have provided a link to this study at the end of the booklet, it is a wonderful read and the research the scientists cite has convinced me that listening to music isn't just something nice to do if I have time, it can be a part of my core wellness practices along with massage, acupuncture, exercise and meditation.

Swollen, Bloated and Puffy

Favorite Slow Tempo, Wordless Music

_____

_____

_____

Positive Emotions and Your Immune System

I had the opportunity to go skydiving first time last year. I felt very scared two days prior to the jump. What was I thinking! I was training to run a half marathon with Team in Training San Diego, why would I risk all that and potentially sprain my ankle landing wrong in a skydiving accident?

It was a beautiful, clear day and we drove out to the facility, went through the check in process and were fitted for our harnesses. When I met my instructor I still didn't know what to expect. I was feeling a little nervous energy, which I let out by chattering and making funny jokes. When I felt the relaxed, confident energy of my instructor, I realized that I was going to be safe and taken care of. I could enjoy the experience instead of becoming overwhelmed by the adrenaline in my body.

Swollen, Bloated and Puffy

Maybe its because of my meditation practice and maybe its because of all my long distance running, but as I prepared to exit the plane, I didn't feel any fear, just curiosity. I remember crouching on the edge of the open door and looking at the Earth below and just knowing how beautiful and striking it was. As I fell, I was caught in a stream of a thousand dreams. I had felt awe on a grand scale.

Research found that showed that those who experience more positive emotions, including feelings of "awe, wonder and amazement" have reduced levels of the cytokine Interleukin 6, a marker of inflammation (Anwar, 2015). Balancing the demands of work, family and social obligations can lead to overflowing to-do lists, a feeling of busyness that leads to anxiety, and the sense of not having enough time to do everything. Taking time to go out in nature and ideally experience awe is one natural way to combat stress. Have you ever seen something amazing and you feel like time literally stood still? That's the beauty of a feeling called awe.

Here's a quick 7 step experiment that can show you the effect of awe on your own body.

Swollen, Bloated and Puffy

1. Take a moment to sit comfortably in a safe space and close your eyes
2. Take a slow, deep breath
3. Bring to mind a time when you experienced awe
4. How did it make you feel, where were you and who were you with? Really feel the emotion in your body
5. Notice where you felt the emotion. Did you shoulders and face relax as you remembered your experience?
6. Open your eyes and take another deep breath
7. How busy and overwhelmed do you feel now versus before you closed your eyes?

Remembering an experience of awe is getting just a glimpse of the positive effects that regular time outdoors in nature can provide.

Things that Make Me Feel Awe, Wonder or Amazement

_____

_____

_____

Swollen, Bloated and Puffy

Laughter can balance the immune system

If you are a friend of mine, you know one of the top five words that describe me could be the word cackle. I absolutely love to laugh. And by laugh, I mean laugh at my own jokes, do silly dances, and hyperventilate just trying to retell a funny story. Bennett & Lengacher (2009) put together an insightful overview of research on the link between humor and immunity. Just smiling or thinking funny thoughts aren't enough to boost immunity and Natural Killer cells, we have got to laugh out loud to reap the positive benefits of humor (Bennett & Lengacher, 2009). If you need an immune boost, add laughter to your life.

Friendship and Your Immune System

Did you know that having friends can make you less likely to contract an upper respiratory illness? A study published in the Journal of the American Medical Association really changed my mind about the value of friendship during cold & flu season. I had previously thought that hanging out with people made it MORE likely that I would catch a cold or flu from them. Research has instead shown that the more robust and

Swollen, Bloated and Puffy

varied your social ties are, the less likely you are to contract a cold (Cohen et al, 1997). Your friends can literally help build your immune system!

One thing that is essential to staying friends with others and ourselves is forgiveness. Researchers have also found that the act of forgiveness can improve immune system function on those with a compromised immune system, leading to a higher percentage of CD4 cells in the total number of lymphocytes in the blood (Harrison, 2011). Forgiveness is Pearl 77 of Dr. Guarneri's *108 Pearls to Awaken Your Healing Potential* and she has some wonderful insights on it in her book (Guarneri, 2017).

Your Favorite Ways to Balance the Immune System:

_____

_____

_____

Swollen, Bloated and Puffy

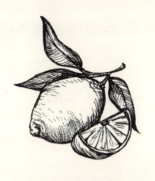

CHAPTER 8

SEVEN TIPS FOR BOOSTING YOUR MOOD AND REDUCING STRESS

I love Gabrielle Bernstein (check her out at GabbyBernstein.com). I first saw her at a Deepak Chopra meditation event at his center in Carlsbad a few years ago. She is so full of positive energy, and she inspires me to keep on using manifesting to put myself into a positive headspace. When I do use manifesting, it definitely draws opportunities into my life. And yet … sometimes I still wake up very shaken and I do still have fears that I will not be successful. I realized recently that I had these doubts – thoughts that I'm not good enough or that things weren't going to come to fruition – in one way or another, for the last 25 years.

With great self-compassion, I'm beginning to realize that comparing my journey to others is a part of my life, not just a phase we go through as teenagers and young adults. Now that I'm in my 40's I wonder if today's society isn't a worse environment for self-doubt than it was before the advent of social media. Back when I was a teenager, all I had to compare myself to were the other kids at my high school. Some of the girls were really pretty, but we all had flaws. In 2017, I am bombarded online with two types of messages – perfectly posed photos on Instagram and snide, judgemental takedowns of people in the comments on Twitter and news articles on Facebook. Have I internalized the message that I need to always put my best foot forward or suffer the wrath of strangers? Should I really be comparing myself to images that took a dozen takes and a filter to create?

I know that being under constant stress hampers the effectiveness of the immune system. Gaining this perspective on the reality of social media has helped me not to stress so much about what I see as I scroll on my tablet or smartphone. What else can we do to weave little stress-busting moments into our day? I have started to compile a list, please email me your ideas at solacesandiego@gmail.com

Swollen, Bloated and Puffy

Ask a child to tell you a joke — you'll get to spend some time with a child's infectious positive energy and share a laugh.

Go for a walk — fresh air and stretch of the legs in nature can energize the body and spirit, especially after staring at a computer screen all day.

Watch cat videos — there's a reason they are so popular on YouTube. Cat lovers find that watching videos of cats brightens their mood.

Give yourself an ear massage — hold one ear in each hand and gently massage the front and back side of each ear, then pull the earlobe gently a few times. Massage little circles with your fingertips on the cheek in front of each ear as well as behind the ear on the neck.

Turn your top fear into a positive outcome. For example, if you are worried about an upcoming meeting, repeat to yourself "I am participating confidently in the meeting and people appreciate my input. I feel comfortable and in control." Repeat silently for 30 seconds each time a fearful thought about the situation strikes.

Swollen, Bloated and Puffy

Close your eyes and try to pick out three different sounds. Reorient yourself away from stressful thoughts and situations by focusing on your sense of hearing.

Smell your favorite flowers. Jasmine and Rose can bring happy feelings – use whole flowers or the essential oils diluted with water in a spray bottle. Some people also love citrus scents, like lemon or orange. Just smelling essential oils may also have a positive effect on stress. Research by Fukada et al (2012) found that inhaling a type of Rose oil reduces stress-induced disruption of the skin barrier because it inhibits the hypothalmo-pituitary-adrenocortical axis (HPA axis) (Fukada, 2012).

Your favorite ways to reduce stress:

_____
_____
_____

Swollen, Bloated and Puffy

IF YOU ARE NERVOUS BEFORE SURGERY

"Basal Cell Carcinoma."

Those three words spoken by my dermatologist last year as she shined a bright light and peered at my right cheek felt like loose sand being stolen from under my feet by an undertow.

"I'll take a biopsy to make sure."

Carcinoma, I thought dully. Carcinoma. Both my parents had died from cancer, so I knew what the word meant.

I had skin cancer.

The next ten minutes: scraping of the pimple that had never healed on my cheek, then an explanation of how I would book surgery went over my head. I asked if it would be written on a sheet of paper—"I'm just not thinking clearly right now." My Derm smiled, "Yes."

Swollen, Bloated and Puffy

I didn't know that that sheet was just the beginning of the paper trail that cancer created. Even a simple skin cancer, the 'no big deal,' the 'we get hundreds of cases a month it's just surgery' type of cancer.

It was decided—I would get an outpatient procedure, booked in the late afternoon, an operation called Mohs surgery. No chemotherapy, no radiation.

One day I would have cancer, the next I wouldn't.

Maybe I would have been fine and maybe I would have been as relaxed as other people who take a small operation like this one in stride. Maybe.

But I made one big mistake—I Googled Mohs Surgery. I waited until it was late at night, after my concerned, loving husband had gone to sleep and I searched on YouTube for "Mohs surgery cheek." That's when the anxiety started, an empty levitating heaviness in the pit of my stomach and pressing tightness in my heart.

All I could think of was being permanently disfigured.

Swollen, Bloated and Puffy

Instead of imagining a healthy recovery, I was mentally preparing myself for the worst—and giving myself a huge case of anxiety.

I have had both really good operations and much more traumatic surgery experiences, and I spent time last year thinking deeply about what happened differently in each situation to make my experience so different.

I had reconstructive surgery almost a decade ago after a skiing accident and felt completely at ease because I intuitively had positive thoughts about my recovery. In contrast, the 2016 surgery to remove skin cancer from my face didn't go so well because I spent time looking at worst-case scenario YouTube videos instead of thinking positively.

Whenever I have a traumatic experience, I try to find a way to use it positively to help others. After my surgery and recovery had been underway, I searched for the answers I didn't find before my operation—how can people facing surgery reduce anxiety and keep their mind focused on healing?

Swollen, Bloated and Puffy

I was very fortunate to find Peggy Huddleston's *Prepare for Surgery, Heal Faster* book earlier this year. Huddleston's method of focusing on positive imagery before surgery has resulted in patients reducing their anxiety levels before surgery and using less pain medication and recovering faster after their operation. The power of focusing on personalized positive imagery has been documented in research studies at the Lahey Clinic (Tufts University Medical School), New England Baptist Hospital (Tufts University Medical School) and Beth Israel Deaconess Medical Center (Harvard Medical School).

After reading her book, I jumped at the chance to train with Huddleston personally and I now offer a workshop in San Diego based on the methods and research in Peggy Huddleston's Prepare for Surgery, Heal Faster book. This one hour program provides San Diegans facing surgery with many of the tools we need to use personalized positive imagery to help reduce anxiety before an operation.

I know how anxiety-provoking surgery can be. Invest an hour of your time to learn how to use personalized positive imagery, family and friends and your surgical team to improve your recovery from plastic, orthopedic or reconstructive surgery in San Diego.

To find a list of upcoming workshops, visit http://www.solacesandiego.com/sandiegolymphaticmassage

Integrative Cardiologist Dr. Mimi Guarneri also recommends mental preparation for surgery. She recommends a pre-surgery hypnosis session and has a hypnotherapist on staff at Pacific Pearl, her center in La Jolla. Find out more here: http://pacificpearllajolla.com/

Music can also have beneficial effects on recovering after surgery. Should you bring music with you to the hospital to enjoy after your surgery? Decide for yourself after reading 'The Neurochemistry of Music' research article here: https://danielevitin.com/levitinlab/articles/2013-TICS_1180.pdf

IMPORTANT POINT: If you feel suddenly anxious after surgery and feel like you cannot catch your breath, please visit the Emergency Room IMMEDIATELY and contact your surgeon. These can be symptoms of a pulmonary embolism.

Swollen, Bloated and Puffy

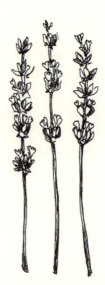

Lavender

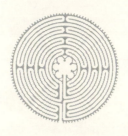

CONCLUSION

The Bottom Line: Live a Healthier Life

OK, so if you've gotten this far, I've thrown a bunch of tips for hacking just about every part of your life except diet to reduce swelling and improve your immune system (research FODMAPS if you want to learn about how diet may affect bloating). I want to sum up my feelings on being healthy. For me, the word healthy describes a level of complete physical, mental and social well-being in an individual.

I want to share with you a list of tough questions I ask myself to take a good, hard look at my life and get a sense of how healthy I am.

Are you able to do all the activities you want to, like run around with the kids after work, or are you so run-down that most evenings are spent on the couch and most mornings are a struggle to get out of bed? Take a moment to relax your forehead, jaw and shoulders. How much tension are you holding in your body day after day?

Mental well-being is at risk in our overstimulated, always-on world. Can you remember people's names? Have you experienced arriving at a destination having no idea how you got there? Have you said something you regret because you react to situations before you have a chance to take a breath and consider your response?

Social well-being is changing as our interactions become more digital. Do you give people you love half your attention because you are also concentrating on social media? Do you feel alone in a group when everyone else is texting? When is the last time you had a deep, meaningful hug?

I have seen many of these signs in myself. The crazy thing is, I find myself making excuses as to why it's OK to feel so tired, overstimulated and distracted. It is amazing how much of life we let pass us by because we are too tired to experience it. Meditation has been a powerful practice in my life. I find that I am more present and can remember names better, respond to situations instead of reacting to them and I have many more moments of awareness during the day where I am able to focus on tasks without getting distracted by my thoughts. If these things concern you, consider taking a meditation class.

The downside of learning to meditate is that I am much more aware of being distracted when I am on social media with friends and loved ones. I am still taking baby steps to reduce my smartphone usage when I am with friends or occupied with other tasks.

Here are my three tips for being more calm and centered:

One: Calm, centered women are aware and accepting when they are not calm and centered. Our quick-fix society puts an emphasis on immediately eliminating any emotion that is not positive. A crying child is distracted with treats or told to 'quiet down,' and a teenager with test anxiety is reassured with 'don't worry, you'll do fine.' It is difficult to have an emotion without trying to change it if it is unwanted or hold on tight to it if it is wanted. We can try it ourselves with this test right now: Wherever we are, try to become aware of our posture and feel our neck, shoulders and back without immediately straightening up or moving around. It's hard to resist! Cultivating an acceptance of our emotions, good and bad, can take away the stress of trying to be someone we are not.

Greater awareness is another key to feeling more centered. As anyone who has snapped "I'm not angry!" to their spouse has realized, knowing when we are irritated is not always easy.

Two: 'Waking up' to our emotions as they happen is developed by the second thing calm, centered women do – meditate. Calm, centered women protect and nurture their daily meditation practice. Research shows that many benefits can be seen after meditating just a few minutes a day (Flaxman & Flook, n.d). The hard part? Finding time and motivation to make meditation a habit. Calm, centered women have found the key to keeping meditation in our daily wellness practices, right along with must-dos like brushing our teeth. The key to making meditation into a habit is to find a 'reminder' that reminds us to meditate. Reserve time for meditation at the same place in our schedules each morning and it will become the automatic thing to do after making a cup of tea or walking the dog.

Three: Calm, centered women take time for mindfulness throughout our day. When we sense ourselves becoming agitated, breathing slowly in and out for thirty seconds or noticing the feeling of our feet on the ground helps us become centered and aware of the present moment. I have used these 'stealth' mindfulness exercises before taking an exam, in the middle of a meeting with colleagues, in my doctor's office in Carmel Valley, at a noisy party or walking down the street in downtown San Diego Gaslamp district, all times where emotions and anxiety can run high.

I hope all these tips help you to reduce swelling and improve your immune system, whether you are dealing with lymphedema, lipedema or the swelling that comes after orthopedic, reconstructive and plastic surgery.

Please email me with any question and especially tips that have worked for you at solacesandiego@gmail.com and please share this booklet with a friend.

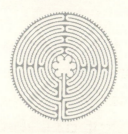

BIBLIOGRAPHY

6 Best Fixes for Pain and Swelling in Your Feet and Ankles. (2016, July 19). Retrieved June 02, 2017, from https://health.clevelandclinic.org/2016/06/6-best-ways-relieve-swollen-feet-ankles-home/

7 Best and Worst Home Remedies for Your Hemorrhoids. (2016, June 03). Retrieved from https://health.clevelandclinic.org/2016/06/7-best-worst-home-remedies-hemorrhoids/

Adults Demonstrate Modified Immune Response After Receiving Massage, Cedars-Sinai Researchers Show. (2010, September 7). Retrieved May 20, 2017, from https://www.cedars-sinai.edu/About-Us/News/News-Releases-2010/Adults-Demonstrate-Modified-Immune-Response-After-Receiving-Massage-Cedars-Sinai-Researchers-Show.aspx

Anwar, Y. (2015, February 2). Add nature, art and religion to life's best anti-inflammatories. Retrieved from http://news.berkeley.edu/2015/02/02/anti-inflammatory/

Battaglia, S. (2003). *The complete guide to aromatherapy* (2nd ed.). Brisbane: International Centre of Holistic Aromatherapy.

Bennett, M. P., & Lengacher, C. (2009). Humor and Laughter May Influence Health IV. Humor and Immune Function. *Evidence-Based Complementary and Alternative Medicine : eCAM*, 6(2), 159–164. http://doi.org/10.1093/ecam/nem149 Retrieved from https://www.ncbi.nlm.nih.gov/pmc/articles/PMC2686627/

Buford, G. (2016) *Eat, Drink, Heal.* Createspace. Find out more at:

http://www.beautybybuford.com/author-dr-gregory-buford/eat-drink-heal-book/

Chanda, M. & Levitin, D. (2013). "Neurochemistry and music."

Trends in Cognitive Sciences , Volume 17 , Issue 4 , 179 – 193. Retrieved from https://daniellevitin.com/levitinlab/articles/2013-TICS_1180.pdf

Cohen S, Doyle WJ, Skoner DP, Rabin BS, Gwaltney JM Jr., "Social ties and susceptibility to the common cold." JAMA. 1997 Jun 25;277(24):1940-4. PMID: 9200634 Retrieved at http://jamanetwork.com/journals/jama/article-abstract/417085

Courtney, R. (2009). The functions of breathing and its dysfunctions and their relationship to breathing therapy. International Journal of Osteopathic Medicine 12(3). https://doi.org/10.1016/j.ijosm.2009.04.002 Retrieved from https://www.researchgate.net/publication/228637154_The_functions_of_breathing_and_its_dysfunctions_and_their_relationship_to_breathing_therapy

Cushing syndrome. (n.d.). Retrieved from http://www.mayoclinic.org/diseases-conditions/cushing-syndrome/home/ovc-20197169

Steffi Dreha-Kulaczewski, Arun A. Joseph, Klaus-Dietmar Merboldt, Hans-Christoph Ludwig, Jutta Gärtner, Jens Frahm, "Inspiration Is the Major Regulator of Human CSF Flow." Journal of Neuroscience 11 February 2015, 35 (6) 2485-2491; DOI: 10.1523/JNEUROSCI.3246-14.2015 Retrieved from http://www.jneurosci.org/content/35/6/2485

Ehrlich, S. (2016, April 1). Edema. Retrieved, from http://umm.edu/health/medical/altmed/condition/edema

Flaxman, G., & Flook, L. (n.d.). Brief Summary of Mindfulness Research. Retrieved from http://marc.ucla.edu/workfiles/pdfs/marc-mindfulness-research-summary.pdf

Freeman, G. (n.d.). Inflammation and Stiffness: The Hallmarks of Arthritis. Retrieved from http://www.arthritis.org/about-arthritis/understanding-arthritis/arthritis-swelling-and-stiffness.php

Fukada M, Kano E, Miyoshi M, et al. "Effect of "rose essential oil" inhalation on stress-induced skin-barrier disruption in rats and humans" Chem Senses. 2012 May; 37(4):347-56. Retrieved from https://www.ncbi.nlm.nih.gov/pubmed/22167272

Guarneri, M. (2017). *108 pearls to awaken your healing potential: a cardiologist translates the science of health and healing into practice*. Carlsbad, CA: Hay House, Inc.

How Sleep Clears the Brain. (2013, October 28). Retrieved from https://www.nih.gov/news-events/nih-research-matters/how-sleep-clears-brain

Jefferson CD; Drake CL, Scofield HM et al. "Sleep hygiene practices in a population-based sample of insomniacs," SLEEP 2005;28(5):611- 615. Retrieved from http://www.journalsleep.org/articles/280509.pdf

Kahn, L. (n.d.). Aromatherapy & Essential Oils to Support the Lymphatic System » Beauty Kliniek Aromatherapy Day Spa & Wellness Center. Retrieved from https://www.beautykliniek.com/aromatherapy-essential-oils-support-lymphatic-system/

MacDonald, G. (2005). *Massage for the hospital patient and medically frail client.* Philadelphia: Lippincott Williams & Wilkins.

Ojeh N, Stojadinovic O, Pastar I, Sawaya A, Yin N, Tomic-Canic M., "The Effects of Caffeine on Wound Healing," Int Wound J. 2016 Oct;13(5):605-13. doi: 10.1111/iwj.12327. Epub 2014 Jul 8. Retrieved at https://www.ncbi.nlm.nih.gov/pubmed/25041108

Owen, A., Haywood, D., & Toussaint, L. (2011). Forgiveness and immune functioning in people living with HIV-AIDS. Washington DC: Paper presented at the Society of Behavioral Medicine. J Relig Health (2014) 53:1317–1328 1327 12 Retrieved at http://www.sbm.org/

meeting/2011/presentations/saturday/paper_sessions/Paper%20Session%2021%20-%20Forgiveness%20and%20immune%20functioning.pdf

Phillips, S. M., Lloyd, G. R., Awick, E. A., and McAuley, E. (2016) Relationship between self-reported and objectively measured physical activity and subjective memory impairment in breast cancer survivors: role of self-efficacy, fatigue and distress. Psycho-Oncology, doi: 10.1002/pon.4156. Retrieved from http://onlinelibrary.wiley.com/doi/10.1002/pon.4156/full

Poor Sleep Quality Increases Inflammation, Community Study Finds. (2010, November 15). Retrieved at http://shared.web.emory.edu/whsc/news/releases/2010/11/poor-sleep-quality-increases-inflammation-study-finds.html

Qaseem A, Wilt TJ, McLean RM, Forciea MA, for the Clinical Guidelines Committee of the American College of Physicians. Noninvasive Treatments for Acute, Subacute, and Chronic Low Back Pain: A Clinical Practice Guideline From the American College of Physicians. Ann Intern Med. 2017;166:514-530. doi: 10.7326/M16-2367 Retrieved from http://annals.org/aim/article/2603228/noninvasive-treatments-acute-subacute-chronic-low-back-pain-clinical-practice

Reynolds, G. (2009, October 14). Phys Ed: Does Exercise Boost Immunity? Retrieved from https://well.blogs.nytimes.com/2009/10/14/phys-ed-does-exercise-boost-immunity/

Rogers, C., Larkey, L. K., & Keller, C. (2009). A Review of Clinical Trials of Tai Chi and Qigong in Older Adults. *Western Journal of Nursing Research*, *31*(2), 245–279. http://doi.org/10.1177/0193945908327529

Retrieved from https://www.ncbi.nlm.nih.gov/pmc/articles/PMC2810462/

Saint Louis, C. (2010, December 15). Wildly Abrasive. Retrieved from http://www.nytimes.com/2010/12/16/fashion/16Skin.html

Sanders, M. L. (2013, September 06). Think Like a Doctor: The Gymnast's Big Belly Solved. Retrieved from https://well.blogs.nytimes.com/2013/09/06/think-like-a-doctor-the-gymnasts-big-belly-solved/

Sassy Water: A Flat Belly Diet Staple. (2011, November 3). Retrieved May 19, 2017, from http://www.prevention.com/weight-loss/flat-belly-diet/flat-belly-diet-and-sassy-water

Shanbhag, V. K. L. (2017). Oil pulling for maintaining oral hygiene – A review. *Journal of Traditional and Complementary Medicine*, 7(1), 106–109. http://doi.org/10.1016/j.jtcme.2016.05.004 Retrieved from https://www.ncbi.nlm.nih.gov/pmc/articles/PMC5198813/

Simcox LE, Ormesher L, Tower C, Greer IA., "Pulmonary thrombo-embolism in pregnancy: diagnosis and management," Breathe (Sheff). 2015 Dec;11(4):282-9. doi: 10.1183/20734735.008815. Retrieved at https://www.ncbi.nlm.nih.gov/pmc/articles/PMC4818214/pdf/EDU-0088-2015.pdf

Starkey, J. (2015, January 26). The Truth About Dry Brushing and What It Does for You. Retrieved from https://health.clevelandclinic.org/2015/01/the-truth-about-dry-brushing-and-what-it-does-for-you/

Stea S, Beraudi A, & De Pasquale D, "Essential Oils for Complementary Treatment of Surgical Patients: State of the Art," Evidence-Based Complementary and Alternative Medicine, vol. 2014, Article ID 726341, 6 pages, 2014. doi:10.1155/2014/726341 Retrieved at https://www.hindawi.com/journals/ecam/2014/726341/

Subramanian RK, PRD, PS., "Alternate Nostril Breathing at Different Rates and its Influence on Heart Rate Variability in Non Practitioners of Yoga." J Clin Diagn Res. 2016 Jan;10(1):CM01-2. doi: 10.7860/JCDR/2016/15287.7094. Epub 2016 Jan 1 Retrieved at https://www.ncbi.nlm.nih.gov/pmc/articles/PMC4740589/

Vitko H, Sekula K & Schreiber M. "Probiotics for Trauma Patients: Should We Be Taking a Precautionary Approach?" J Trauma Nurs 24 (1), 46-52. Jan-Feb 2017. DOI: 10.1097/JTN.0000000000000263 Retrieved from https://www.ncbi.nlm.nih.gov/labs/articles/28033143/

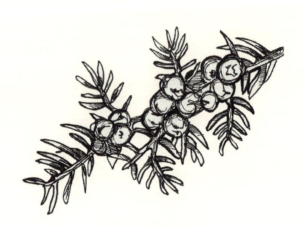

Juniper

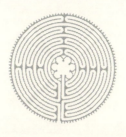

ABOUT THE AUTHOR

Kathleen Lisson is Board Certified in Therapeutic Massage and Bodywork and is a Certified Lymphedema Therapist. She owns Solace Massage and Mindfulness and has taught classes at IPSB Massage College in San Diego.

Kathleen holds a Bachelors of Applied Science in Massage Therapy, is an NHI (Natural Healing Institute of Naturopathy) Certified Aromatherapist, a MMI (McLean Meditation Institute) Certified Meditation Teacher and is certified to present Peggy Huddleston's 'Prepare for Surgery, Heal Faster' workshop.

After 14 years in a high-stress career in public relations for the New York State legislature, she began her second career as a massage therapist at the nonprofit Adams Avenue Integrative Health,

About the Author

where she partnered with naturopaths, chiropractors and acupuncturists to provide care to families in the Normal Heights neighborhood in San Diego. She has also volunteered to provide free chair massage to underserved communities in City Heights at Tubman-Chavez Center and the East African Cultural Community Center through the nonprofit Alternative Healing Network.

Kathleen is the author of articles published in the Elephant Journal and the Labyrinth Pathways 10th edition. She has been quoted in the Prevention Magazine November 2016 issue and online in Bustle, Consumer Reports, Massage Magazine, Prevention and Runner's World.

Social Media:

http://www.solacesandiego.com

https://www.facebook.com/SolaceSanDiego

https://www.instagram.com/kathleenlisson/